The British Medical Association
FAMILY DOCTOR GUIDE *to*
ASTHMA

D0101050

The British Medical Association

FAMILY DOCTOR GUIDE *to*

ASTHMA

PROFESSOR JON AYRES

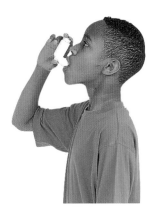

MEDICAL EDITOR
DR. TONY SMITH

DORLING KINDERSLEY
LONDON • NEW YORK • SYDNEY • MOSCOW
www.dk.com

IMPORTANT

PLEASE NOTE

A DORLING KINDERSLEY BOOK
www.dk.com

Senior Editor Mary Lindsay
Senior Designer Sarah Hall
Project Editor David Tombesi-Walton
Designer Laura Watson
DTP Designer Jason Little
Production Controller Michelle Thomas

Managing Editor Stephanie Jackson
Managing Art Editor Nigel Duffield

Produced for Dorling Kindersley Limited by
Design Revolution, Queens Park Villa,
30 West Drive, Brighton, East Sussex BN2 2GE.
Editorial Manager Ian Whitelaw
Art Director Fiona Roberts
Editor Julie Whitaker
Designer Vanessa Good

Published in Great Britain in 1999 by
Dorling Kindersley Limited,
9 Henrietta Street, London WC2E 8PS

2 4 6 8 10 9 7 5 3 1

A CIP catalogue record for this book is available from the British Library

ISBN 0 7513 0676 2

Reproduced by Colourscan, Singapore
Printed in Hong Kong by Wing King Tong

Contents

What is asthma?

Most people would recognise asthma in a child or adult as attacks of wheezy breathlessness, sometimes on exertion, sometimes at rest, sometimes mild, sometimes severe. Some would recognise specific 'triggers' – for example, animals, fumes, pollens.

Some might think of asthma as a condition of children, some as a condition able to affect someone of any age. Some would regard it as an occasional nuisance requiring intermittent treatment only, others as a persistent, significant problem needing continuous treatment. Surely they can't all be right?

In a way they can, although it is this wide range of factors involved in asthma that makes it extremely difficult to come up with a simple definition.

The word 'asthma' is used as a blanket term to cover a condition that is characterised by episodes of breathlessness caused by intermittent narrowing of the bronchial tubes – or airways – within the lung. There are many factors that contribute to the development of asthma in the first instance and many that can induce attacks. In addition, these will vary from individual to individual.

ASTHMA SYMPTOMS
A common symptom of asthma is wheezing, which is often accompanied by chest tightness and breathlessness.

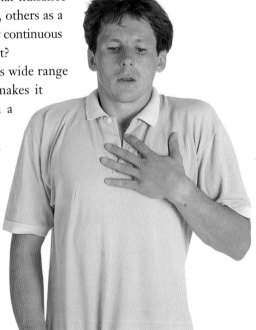

7

The Respiratory System

The airways (trachea, bronchi and bronchioles) and airspaces within the lungs supply oxygen to and remove carbon dioxide from the body. Mucus is moved through the lungs by cilia (tiny hairs) on the airways' internal walls.

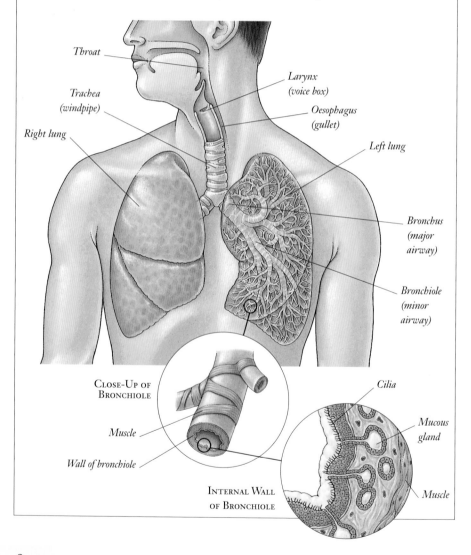

Throat

Trachea
(windpipe)

Larynx
(voice box)

Oesophagus
(gullet)

Right lung

Left lung

Bronchus
(major
airway)

Bronchiole
(minor
airway)

CLOSE-UP OF
BRONCHIOLE

Cilia

Muscle

Mucous
gland

Wall of bronchiole

INTERNAL WALL
OF BRONCHIOLE

Muscle

The best definition is that asthma is a condition in which the airways within the lung are inflamed and so are more sensitive to specific factors (triggers) that cause the airways to narrow, reducing airflow through them and making the individual breathless and/or wheezy.

This sensitivity of the airways enjoys the medical label 'bronchial hyper-reactivity'. In the surgery or clinic doctors use the term 'twitchy tubes'!

So asthma is not one disease: it covers a multitude of different patterns. Like the word 'cancer' it tells you roughly what sort of condition we are dealing with, what ballpark we are in. Under that general heading you will find a range of severities, a range of triggering factors and a range of outcomes. It logically follows that what is good for one asthmatic person may be unsuitable for another.

Asthma is a very individual condition and management needs to be personalised because of the variety of factors that underlie each individual's asthma.

KEY POINTS

- Because of the wide range of factors involved in causing asthma and the variety of responses the body's airways make, it is not easy to define asthma simply.
- Asthma is not one disease. Like the word 'cancer' it covers a multitude of different patterns.

How much asthma is there?

The short answer is – a lot! Up-to-date estimates suggest that 20 per cent of children of primary school age and around 6–7 per cent of the general population in the United Kingdom suffer from asthma.

Asthma is the most common condition to be found in Western populations, affecting over three million individuals in England and Wales alone. In children, boys are twice as frequently affected as girls, while in adult life the condition is slightly more common among women.

▪ IS ASTHMA INCREASING? ▪

Asthma has increased over the past two decades, regardless of what measure of asthma you look at. For example, between the mid-1970s and the early 1990s, there was around a five-fold increase in the numbers of patients coming to their GP with an attack of asthma, particularly in children. There was also an increase in hospital admissions up to the early 1990s, again particularly in children, possibly reflecting the fact

CHILDHOOD ASTHMA
Asthma in children appears to be on the increase; up to 20 per cent of the school-age population are believed to have asthmatic symptoms.

that parents are more likely to seek medical advice for their children than for themselves, although other factors are also likely to play a part. Gratifyingly, the rise stopped in the early 1990s and has fallen slightly since.

WHY DID ASTHMA INCREASE?

It is possible that some of the increase is due to doctors now using the word 'asthma' whereas before they would have used 'wheezy bronchitis', but this cannot explain the greater part of the rise. Exposure to allergens in the home, viral infections, aspects of the indoor environment such as central heating, air pollution, the stress of modern living – even the treatments used for asthma itself – have all been blamed for the increase. However, evidence for any of these individually being responsible is limited. In fact, it is highly likely that the rise is due to a combination of these factors although allergies are likely to be the more important cause.

DEATHS FROM ASTHMA

Fortunately, death from asthma is not common. In the mid-1960s a short-lived epidemic of deaths caused by asthma occurred which some thought might be the result of a toxic effect of one of the asthma inhalers on sale at the time. This has been disputed over the years and other factors may have been of importance; it is unlikely that we shall ever know the complete story surrounding that event.

In fact, most deaths from asthma are caused by the undertreatment of patients, and it has been shown that two-thirds of asthma deaths would have been preventable with adequate treatment. Lately, there has been a further slight rise in asthma deaths in patients over the age of 50 although this, again, settled down in the 1990s. Why this has occurred is not clear, although in the older patient differentiating between asthma and chronic bronchitis is often difficult and this may have led to a change in diagnostic fashion.

ASTHMA-FREE POPULATIONS

Although asthma appears to be on the increase in many countries, there are places in the world where it is rare. For example, asthma rarely occurs among the Eskimo population of North America, probably because the harsh climate is not hospitable to the house dust mite.

GEOGRAPHICAL DIFFERENCES

There are certainly some parts of the UK where asthma admissions and GP attendances are more common and other areas where they are less so. However, the differences are modest and do not form a clear-cut geographical pattern, unlike attacks of acute bronchitis, which are higher in the north, becoming less so towards the south. Although the differences within the UK are slight, there are quite huge differences in the distribution of asthma in different parts of the world. It is almost unheard of in Eskimos and black Africans living in rural areas, whereas in the Western Caroline Islands nearly 50 per cent of the inhabitants have asthma, with three-quarters of children being affected.

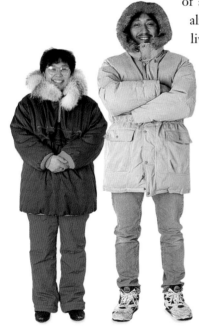

Between these extremes are the westernised populations such as people in the UK and other European countries, Australia and New Zealand, which all have roughly the same amount of asthma. Interestingly, those parts of the world with less asthma are those that are less encouraging to the survival of the house dust mite.

KEY POINTS

- Over three million individuals in England and Wales alone have asthma.
- Boys are more frequently affected than girls, but the condition is slightly more common in women than in men.

Causes and triggers of asthma

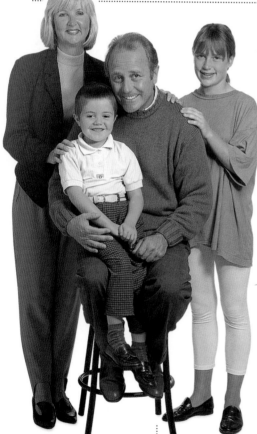

*M*ost people know that asthma can 'run in families' and there is undoubtedly a hereditary component to this condition, particularly in allergic (or extrinsic) asthma. The genetic factor is much less marked in patients where allergy is not involved (intrinsic asthma).

HOW DOES IT START?

The tendency to develop asthma is not absolute: it is not inherited in the way that eye colour and blood group are, and a patient with very severe asthma can have children who never develop the condition.

The role of environmental factors (for example, allergens, exposure to passive smoking) are therefore paramount in the development – and exacerbation – of asthma. Nevertheless, it is clear that, in order for the 'seed' of asthma to germinate, the 'soil' must be right!

A FAMILY CONCERN
Asthma (particularly when an allergen is involved) has a tendency to run in families.

14

HOUSE DUST MITE AND OTHER FACTORS

Against this background, many factors seem to be responsible for the first appearance of the symptoms of asthma. For instance, asthma beginning in adult life often seems to start following a cold or viral infection; alternatively, exposure to a trigger in the workplace may be the initiating factor.

The most important factor in precipitating asthma, however, particularly in children, is exposure to the house dust mite. This little beast, smaller than a pin point, lives in our carpets, mattresses and furry toys. There can be as many as two million in each mattress!

When a susceptible individual is exposed to a protein in the faecal pellet of the house dust mite over a period of time, the body's white cells become sensitive to this 'foreign substance'. As the protein is inhaled, a reaction to it occurs in the lining of the bronchial tubes, resulting in inflammation of the airways. The inflammation makes the lining irritable so that any further exposure, either to the house dust mite or any other potential trigger factor, will result in narrowing of the bronchial tubes and the symptoms of asthma.

There are other things that may be contributory factors to the initiation of asthma. Smoking by the mother during pregnancy and exposure to passive cigarette smoke in childhood may contribute in some cases.

THE HOUSE DUST MITE
The faeces of this mite (magnified here x500), which lives in carpets, mattresses and other soft furnishings, can trigger asthma.

The Development of Asthma

- Inheritance
- Mother smoking during pregnancy
- Passive smoking in childhood
- Allergens (especially the house dust mite)
- Colds or viral infections
- Occupational exposures

15

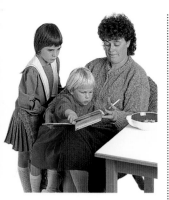

AIRWAY INFLAMMATION

Asthma, then, is due to inflammation, which makes the airways more irritable. Inflammation is the body's attempt to respond to a range of assaults and is seen in many illnesses such as arthritis, colitis and dermatitis. Problems arise for the patient when the inflammation does not resolve and becomes long-standing (or chronic), as is the case in asthma.

The normal airway is lined with a delicate protective layer called the mucosa, or epithelium. This layer consists of various types of cell with different jobs. Some can produce mucus, while others help to clear the mucus from the airway by wafting the secretions up the bronchial tubes via movement of tiny fingers or cilia, which are found on the surface of these cells. These cilia are some of the first structures to be destroyed by cigarette smoke, which also stimulates increased mucus production because the smoke causes inflammation. This is the reason why smokers cough up phlegm. In some patients with asthma, cough is also important and this is hardly surprising now we have seen that asthma is an inflammatory condition.

Below the mucosa, a second layer (the submucosa) lies over a spiral sheet of muscle which, in asthma, contracts when a patient inhales a trigger such as grass pollen.

There are three separate processes which lead to airway narrowing and wheezy breathlessness. Firstly, the middle layer of the airway (submucosa) becomes swollen; secondly, the mucous glands produce more secretions (which have to be coughed up to clear the airways); and thirdly, the smooth muscle contracts as a result of the release of substances from inflammatory cells.

The net result of these three effects is to narrow the airways, making it more difficult to get air in and out – which leads to wheezy breathlessness. Different forms of treatment have been devised which can attack each component of the airway narrowing.

In asthma, symptoms can occur for no obvious reason or may be caused by a clear-cut exposure to a known 'trigger factor' such as grass pollen during the summer. Equally, the airway narrowing can reverse with improvement of symptoms either spontaneously or following the use of a reliever drug. It is this variability that is so characteristic of asthma. We take advantage of this both when making the diagnosis and when devising ways of keeping asthma under control.

How Asthma Affects the Airways

During an asthma attack, the muscle walls of the airways (bronchi and bronchioles) contract, causing their internal diameter to narrow. Increased mucus secretion and inflammation of the airways' inner linings cause further narrowing.

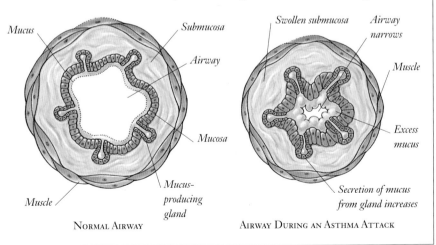

Mucus

Submucosa

Airway

Mucosa

Mucus-producing gland

Muscle

NORMAL AIRWAY

Swollen submucosa

Airway narrows

Muscle

Excess mucus

Secretion of mucus from gland increases

AIRWAY DURING AN ASTHMA ATTACK

CASE HISTORIES

If you have asthma you will recognise that several factors will set off your asthma (see chart on pp.20–21).

Case History 1: CHILDHOOD ASTHMA

John is seven years old and his mother, who had hay fever when younger, had noticed that he had begun to cough when running around in the garden. She had taken him to the GP who had prescribed antibiotics with no benefit on three separate occasions.

The symptoms became more persistent and it was only when he developed wheeze on exertion during a games lesson at school that the penny dropped and a diagnosis of asthma was made. John was prescribed a bronchodilator (tube-opening) inhaler to be used when he has symptoms, since which time he has been well and able to play without getting breathless.

Case History 2: FUR ALLERGY

Caroline, a 27-year-old woman with long-standing asthma, was referred to a chest physician because of worsening symptoms over the previous two months. She was known to have many allergic triggers for her asthma, including grass and tree pollens and a number of furry animals.

As part of the assessment, the doctor visited her at home to be greeted by 14 cats which, it emerged, she bred and showed, a fact of which her GP was unaware.

Caroline had an extremely strong skin test reaction to cat fur but fervently denied that stroking the cats made her worse. It was clear that the cats were a major cause of her continuing asthma, providing a constant exposure to

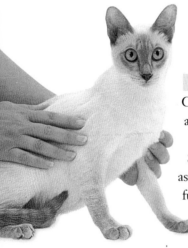

FURRY FRIENDS
Caroline's pet cats proved to be the main cause of her asthma attacks. She was allergic to their fur and dander (the dead skin that they constantly shed).

allergen, which effectively gave her recurrent, virtually continuous asthma episodes. She would not get rid of the cats, her best friends, and a balance has had to be struck between bad asthma caused by exposure to allergens and the benefits of keeping her friends and companions.

Case History 3: PERFUME ALLERGY

Georgina had worked for 22 years in the cosmetic department of the local department store. After a viral infection one autumn, she developed asthma which initially proved easy to treat by the usual means.

However, over a year Georgina developed worsening symptoms, particularly cough, and the main trigger appeared to be scents. She stopped using perfumes herself but, after an initial slight improvement, her symptoms clearly began to relate to her exposure to perfumes at the store. Eventually she had to give up her job (she was 58) and her symptoms improved immeasurably.

PERFUME SENSITIVITY
Georgina's sensitivity to perfumes began many years after she started work at the cosmetic department. Once sensitised, however, she could no longer tolerate contact with scents and had to leave her job.

Case History 4: AIR POLLUTION

David, a severe asthmatic in his 20s, had had some difficulty in controlling his asthma one autumn. He had increased his inhalers and his GP had given him two courses of steroid tablets.

Coming up to Christmas, his asthma at last seemed to be stabilising somewhat, when a five-day air pollution episode hit Birmingham, reaching peak levels on Christmas Eve. By that day David's asthma had become very much worse and, in spite of more steroid tablets and increasing use of his nebuliser, he had to be admitted to hospital – a most unacceptable way to spend Christmas!

Main Trigger Factors in Asthma

In a susceptible person, any of the following triggers can start an asthma attack.
An individual soon recognises which factors affect him or her.

EXERCISE

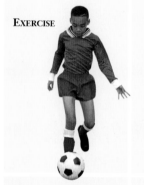

This is a particularly obvious trigger in children, where it may often be the only thing that brings out asthmatic symptoms. The problem is that breathlessness on exertion is often attributed to non-fitness rather than asthma. The schoolboy is then felt to be not fit enough to play as a forward on the football field (putting us in danger of producing a nation of asthmatic goalkeepers!).

ALLERGENS

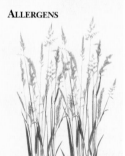

Pollen is the best recognised trigger but animals, particularly cats and horses, are also potent causes of attacks. Chronic exposure may result in more persistent symptoms, and the importance of animals in the house may be missed as the patient claims to be able to stroke the cat without 'getting an attack' not realising that long-term exposure is causing chronic symptoms.

FUMES, DUST AND ODOURS

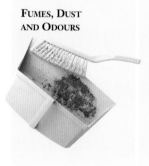

Cigarette smoke is a potent trigger for many patients, as are dusty environments, where the dust acts as an irritant. Odours, such as scent or after-shave, can be a trigger for certain individuals but this is not an allergy. Presumably, it is an irritant reaction to the chemicals involved, and the best treatment is avoidance where possible, although this may have important consequences.

Main Trigger Factors in Asthma (cont'd)

COLDS AND VIRUSES

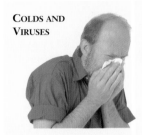

Viral infections are the most common trigger for asthma across the age spectrum. Antibiotics are only effective in treating bacterial infections which are very rare in asthma: viruses are completely unaffected by antibiotics, which have little or no place in the management of asthma yet are prescribed for episodes of worsening asthma.

EMOTIONS AND STRESS

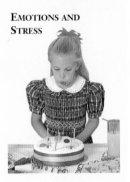

Children often become more wheezy at birthday parties, where the combination of excitement and exertion makes asthma more obvious. Asthma was for years regarded as a neurotic condition, but it is now clear that emotional factors act only as triggers, not initiators, of asthma. Excitement, grief and stress can all trigger an asthma attack.

We have occasionally found patients to have attacks when attending funerals and other such stressful situations.

CLIMATE AND POLLUTION

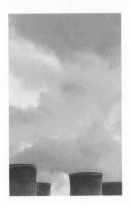

Many patients with asthma know that their condition is affected by the weather, but there is no uniform pattern. Some prefer cold to warm weather; others prefer hot, dry atmospheres. You, the patient, know best and will usually adjust your behaviour and treatment accordingly.

Air pollution episodes are well recognised as causing exacerbations of asthma, particularly in patients with more severe asthma, in both the summer ozone periods and the winter episodes. There is, however, no direct evidence that exposure to air pollution at current levels will turn a non-asthmatic person into an asthmatic patient.

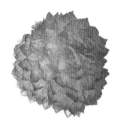

POLLEN GRAIN
Seen here greatly magnified, flower and tree pollen grains can trigger asthma attacks in pollen-sensitive people.

Case History 5: **POLLEN SENSITIVITY**

One summer, a severe thunderstorm struck southern Britain, moving from the Southampton area, up through London and then northwards through East Anglia. During this period hundreds of patients went to casualty departments with attacks of asthma. Many had no idea that they were asthmatic, although most admitted to wheezing with their hay fever (i.e., they had had asthma but had not been told!). It is likely that a specific combination of meteorological factors and high pollen counts was the cause of the outbreak, a rather dramatic example of the weather affecting patients with asthma.

KEY POINTS

- Asthma can run in families, but a patient with quite severe asthma can have children who never develop the condition.
- The most important factor in initiating asthma, particularly in children, is the house dust mite.
- Symptoms may occur for no obvious reason, or may be caused by exposure to one or more trigger factors, such as exercise, viral infection, fumes, dust, grief, stress, climate and pollution.
- Different combinations of trigger factors are important for different patients.

INTERACTING TRIGGER FACTORS

In many cases, two or more of these factors will interact, and different combinations will prove important for different individuals.

Asthma is a very personal condition – what is good for one individual may not necessarily be good for another and patterns of avoidance, treatment and planning in advance need to be organised for each individual person.

Symptoms and diagnosis

Diagnosis of asthma is often difficult as the symptoms can easily be confused with other respiratory complaints. A firm diagnosis may be made after taking a history and undertaking tests.

A REASSURING TEST
Although a physical examination is reassuring, it is less important than tests of lung function.

WHAT ARE THE SYMPTOMS?

Asthma can occur with one or more of four main symptoms: wheeze, breathlessness, cough and chest tightness.

Wheeze and breathlessness are the most well-recognised symptoms, usually coming on intermittently either in response to a recognised trigger or out of the blue. However, breathlessness without wheeze can frequently occur.

One symptom often not recognised as being caused by asthma is cough – either a dry cough or cough with phlegm – which typically occurs at night or on exercise.

Failure to recognise that cough can be caused by asthma often results in a diagnosis of bronchitis being made. Attacks of bronchitis are usually

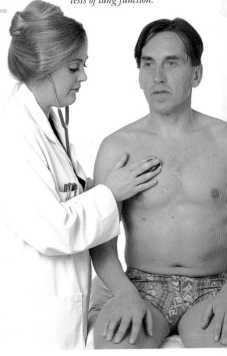

The Four Main Symptoms of Asthma

Wheeze and breathlessness, asthma's most common symptoms, may occur together or separately. Persistent cough is less well recognised, and chest tightness may only be apparent on exertion.

WHEEZE
With or without breathlessness, wheeze may occur in response to a trigger or for no obvious reason.

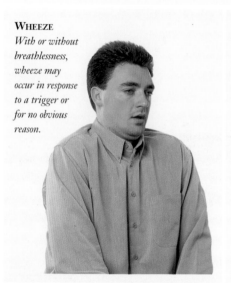

BREATHLESSNESS
Often associated with wheeze and cough, but may also occur alone.

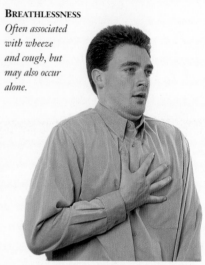

COUGH
A phlegm-producing or a dry cough may be signs of asthma.

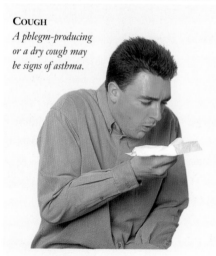

CHEST TIGHTNESS
Although often a symptom of asthma, chest tightness may be mistaken for a heart problem in older people.

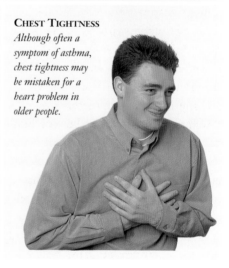

treated by antibiotics, which is a quite inappropriate treatment for asthma. More than two episodes of persistent cough – with or without wheeze or breathlessness – should raise the question of underlying asthma in the minds of both patient and doctor.

The fourth main symptom of asthma is chest tightness. Often, this occurs on exertion and when this happens in an older patient a diagnosis of angina may be made, and it may be quite a difficult problem for the doctor to sort out.

Although the symptoms of asthma often occur for no apparent reason, characteristically they can wake patients and are often a problem on waking in the morning. Waking at night with asthma means that the asthma is being inadequately treated. Exercise, particularly in children, is a frequent trigger for worsening symptoms, often resulting in the child missing games at school.

HOW IS ASTHMA DIAGNOSED?

The trouble with these symptoms is that they occur in many other types of lung – or heart – condition. So, a careful history of what the symptoms are, what sets them off, how long they last, how bad they are and whether there are any recognisable patterns of symptoms, is essential to the doctor in helping him or her arrive at a diagnosis.

Although listening to the chest is part of any examination, very often in asthma it doesn't help the doctor a great deal. The absence of wheezing does NOT mean that asthma isn't the diagnosis!

Conversely, all that wheezes is not asthma – making the diagnosis of asthma quite difficult.

EXERCISE AND ASTHMA
Children with asthma frequently find that exercise can precipitate an attack. However, if the asthma is adequately controlled, it should not be a barrier to sports and other activities.

25

Conditions That Share the Symptoms of Asthma

The symptoms of asthma occur in some other respiratory disorders and a few heart conditions. This table shows in which diseases and how commonly the symptoms are seen.

DIAGNOSIS	WHEEZE	BREATHLESSNESS	COUGH	CHEST TIGHTNESS
Asthma	● ● ●	● ● ●	● ● ●	● ● ●
Chronic bronchitis	● ● ●	● ● ●	● ● ●	● ●
Emphysema	● ●	● ● ●	○	● ● ●
Bronchiectasis	● ●	● ●	● ● ● ●	● ●
Angina	○	● ●	○	● ● ● ●
Heart failure	● ●	● ● ● ●	● ●	● ●

KEY	○ *Symptom not usually seen*	● ● ● *Symptom often seen*
	● ● *Symptom can be seen*	● ● ● ● *Symptom virtually always seen*

BREATHING TESTS

Although a diagnosis of asthma may have been made on history alone, some simple tests are often used to help. In older patients, in whom heart complaints are common, an electrocardiogram (ECG, or heart trace) may help, but breathing tests form the mainstay of asthma investigation.

There are two main types of breathing test used in diagnosing asthma – peak-flow tests and spirometry. Both measure how narrow the airways may be, because the narrower the airways, the slower the flow of air through them, and the lower the readings.

THE PEAK-FLOW METER

The peak-flow meter is a small, cheap and robust instrument and gives an idea of the narrowness of the airways by measuring the maximum, or peak, rate at which air can be expelled. This is the method most likely to be used by GPs as a single reading in the surgery. However, you may be able to use one to measure your peak flow two, three or four times a day to show variation in values over the day. A normal individual will show very little variation in peak flow over days and weeks, whereas an individual with asthma shows either consistent or intermittent variation. A common pattern is the 'morning dip' one, values being lowest on waking. Sometimes the fall in peak flow is intermittent, often in response to a recognised trigger such as cat fur.

Measuring peak flow in this way is particularly helpful if you complain of only intermittent symptoms. Daily peak flow monitoring can be extremely helpful in

Cursor

Scale (litres/ minute)

Mouthpiece

PEAK-FLOW METER
The peak-flow meter is a simple device. After taking a deep breath, the user blows into the mouthpiece. The cursor is moved by the exhaled breath, and the point on the scale at which it comes to rest shows the maximum speed of air flow out of the lungs.

How to Use a Peak-Flow Meter

Your doctor or asthma nurse will show you how to use your peak-flow meter correctly. These instructions are a reminder.

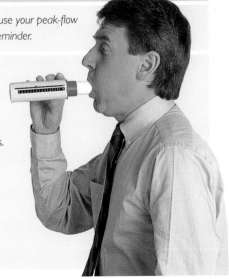

1 Stand up if possible.
2 Check cursor is on zero.
3 Take a deep breath in, place peak-flow meter in the mouth (hold horizontally) and close lips.
4 Blow suddenly and hard.
5 Note number indicated by cursor.
6 Return cursor to zero.
7 Repeat twice to obtain three readings.
8 Write down the best of the three readings.

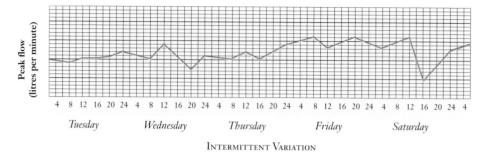

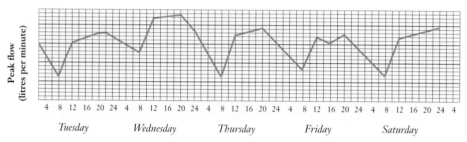

**Peak flow
(litres per minute)**

4 8 12 16 20 24 4 8 12 16 20 24 4 8 12 16 20 24 4 8 12 16 20 24 4 8 12 16 20 24 4

Tuesday   *Wednesday*   *Thursday*   *Friday*   *Saturday*

INTERMITTENT VARIATION

**Peak flow
(litres per minute)**

4 8 12 16 20 24 4 8 12 16 20 24 4 8 12 16 20 24 4 8 12 16 20 24 4 8 12 16 20 24 4

Tuesday   *Wednesday*   *Thursday*   *Friday*   *Saturday*

'MORNING DIP' VARIATION

PEAK FLOW CHARTS

Asthma sufferers frequently show variations in their peak flow readings. These distinctive patterns indicate intermittent variation (top) and the classic 'morning dip' variation (bottom).

management plans by acting as an 'early warning system' to anticipate worsening asthma.

SPIROMETRY

This is mostly used at chest clinics and in hospitals, although an increasing number of general practices now use spirometry. It measures not only how fast air can be blown out but also the amount blown out with each breath. It gives us more information but cannot give us the day-to-day measurements of peak-flow readings.

'REVERSIBILITY' TESTS

Sometimes these breathing tests are performed before and after inhalation of a bronchodilator drug, which opens the airways. If the readings increase by 15 per cent or more after inhaling the drug, the airway narrowing is said to be reversible and confirms a diagnosis of asthma. Even asthmatic patients do not always show reversibility on every occasion tested, but it is nevertheless a very useful diagnostic test in patients in whom asthma is suspected.

OTHER BREATHING TESTS

If your diagnosis is difficult to sort out, you may be sent to a lung function laboratory; here more complicated tests are arranged, usually at the request of a hospital doctor.

KEY POINTS

- The four main symptoms of asthma are wheeze, breathlessness, cough and chest tightness.
- Waking at night with asthma means that the asthma is being inadequately treated.
- More than two episodes of persistent cough should suggest asthma.
- Wheezing does not necessarily indicate asthma, and asthma does not necessarily involve wheezing.
- Breathing tests are often used to help confirm the diagnosis.

Prevention and self-help

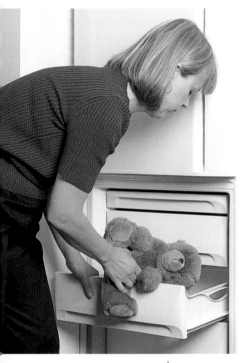

MAKING SOFT TOYS SAFE
Putting soft toys in the
freezer compartment for
12 hours every week will
kill any house dust mites.

Although a diagnosis of asthma may seem to lead inevitably to the use of drugs to control the condition, there are several ways in which you and your family can help reduce symptoms. Equally, there are some environmental modifications that are not believed to be of help.

AVOIDING ALLERGENS

Controlling the house dust mite can be very important in some patients, but the measures are expensive. The use of occlusive bedding is effective but extremely costly unless simple polythene sheeting is used to enclose the mattress and each pillow completely. This makes for a very crinkly and sweaty bed, however! Sprays to kill the mites are ineffective on their own in controlling asthma. In theory, carpets and loose fittings should be removed, and some recommend blinds instead of curtains. Cuddly toys should be put in the deep freeze for 12 hours a week to kill the mites. Because these measures are time-consuming or expensive, inhaled therapy is a much easier method of controlling symptoms for most people.

Getting rid of domestic pets is a contentious issue. Where there is undoubted allergy to cats, dogs or rabbits, a balance has to be struck between control of asthma using inhalers and the grief that can be caused by banishing the pet! Nevertheless, long-term exposure to pets, even those that do not induce an obvious attack, can chronically worsen asthma by exposing a sensitised patient to high levels of allergen. In the more severe asthmatic patient, where control is more difficult, sometimes we have to insist on removal.

I believe that patients' wishes are very important. Some would rather get rid of a pet than use inhalers; others would rather suffer asthma than lose what is often their best friend. Only when beliefs and wishes cause risk to the patient should we be emphatic about parting with the pet.

CENTRAL HEATING

There is no direct evidence one way or the other that any particular form of central heating is either good or bad for patients with asthma. The belief that gas fired central heating dries the air too much has been reported by some patients with asthma, but it is unlikely that this is a major problem. On the other hand, there are good theoretical reasons to believe that ducted or warm air central heating may cause a problem, especially in those patients with allergy to house dust mite. Unfortunately, it is very expensive to

Helping Yourself or Your Child

- Don't smoke cigarettes
- Avoid colds where possible
- Control allergen exposures
- Establish a self-management plan with the help of your doctor
- Keep teachers informed about your child's asthma and the need for access to inhalers on demand
- Where obvious triggers are known, avoid them

replace such systems, especially when there is no guarantee that the patient will improve after removal. I do, however, advise my patients to avoid installing these systems if they are putting in a new one.

BEDROOM TEMPERATURE

A famous doctor of the seventeenth century, Sir John Floyer, himself an asthmatic, believed that when asthma woke a patient up at night this was due to 'the heat of the bed'! Equally, it has been said that sleeping with the bedroom window open, or at least keeping the air cool at night is a help to asthmatics. In truth, there is no clear-cut answer. Some prefer the cooler night air, other people will find it causes them to wheeze more, particularly if they have to get up at night for some other reason. Again, it is up to you to adjust your environment according to what suits you best.

COLDS AND FLU
Respiratory infections, such as the common cold or influenza, can cause asthmatic symptoms to worsen.

VIRAL INFECTIONS

Viruses are an unavoidable cause of worsening asthma but it makes sense to put off a visit to or from someone with a streaming cold! For mums and schoolchildren, however, this is unavoidable – children have to go to school and should not be kept off just because of the risk of catching a cold.

FOOD ALLERGIES

A small proportion of patients with asthma, particularly children, undoubtedly have food sensitivities. Again, a balance has to be struck between the wishes of the patient and control of asthma.

True food allergy is not particularly common but is undoubtedly more common than many doctors believe. The diagnosis is often difficult and involves time-consuming tests. Skin tests can be very misleading and should not be relied upon to diagnose or exclude food allergy. In an important minority, identifying a food or foods that worsen an individual's asthma can have a dramatic effect.

A clear history of, for example, wheezing within minutes of eating a peanut, is easy to recognize, and the best treatment is avoidance. On the other hand, sensitivity to dairy products or wheat is more difficult to recognise because the effects are more chronic and not so dramatic.

Case History 1: NUT ALLERGY

Nick had had asthma since childhood and he had always known that peanuts could cause very severe attacks. He had managed to prevent this by scrupulously avoiding all peanut-containing foods, often a difficult job! During his teens his asthma improved considerably but he still avoided peanuts. On the odd occasion when he took in a mouthful of food containing peanuts he would immediately notice a tingling sensation in his mouth and would spit out the uneaten food. This usually prevented an attack.

One day, while eating a meal at the house of his new girlfriend, he suddenly realised that he had swallowed a mouthful of peanut-containing food. Within minutes, his tongue and lips had swollen and he had begun a severe asthma attack. By the time he reached hospital he was blue and unconscious. Luckily, he got there extremely quickly but he still required ventilation for

A SEVERE REACTION
Within minutes of eating a meal containing nuts, Nick's lips and tongue became swollen, and he quickly lapsed into unconsciousness.

a short period before recovering. His girlfriend and her mother were mortified as they had been unaware of his peanut allergy – one of the food allergies that patients rarely if ever grow out of – thus highlighting the dangers of 'hidden' food allergens.

If you think you are sensitive to certain foods, you should be investigated by a doctor with relevant expertise.

Case History 2: WHEAT ALLERGY

Carolyn was 35 years old and had had asthma since her teens. Initially, it had affected her quality of life but she had managed to develop a career and generally had her asthma under good control. Over a period of two to three years, however, Carolyn began to suffer worsening symptoms and found she was needing frequent courses of oral steroids. Concerned, she asked to be referred to hospital where drug treatment was increased to a maximum without success. She was then admitted to hospital to undergo a food exclusion regimen, which suggested that she might be sensitive to wheat products. When challenged with wheat in capsule form after a period of abstension, her asthma deteriorated over a week, confirming the suspicion. Since avoiding wheat her asthma has been well controlled, although she is still on inhalers at moderate dose, and she has only rarely needed a course of oral steroids.

EXCLUSION DIET
Since eliminating wheat products such as bread from her diet, Carolyn's asthma has been well controlled.

If you are shown to have a problem, avoiding the foods is the only way forward. Avoidance of foods that are not often eaten, like shellfish, is relatively straightforward. However, if you are sensitive to dairy products or wheat – two of the more common recognised problem foodstuffs – the diet may become particularly tiresome and antisocial, especially if your asthma symptoms are modest. Some patients would rather stick to a diet than take any drugs at all. Only rarely will asthma symptoms be completely controlled by dietary means, which should be seen as complementary to adequate medical treatment.

CIGARETTE SMOKE

Cigarette smoke is bad for asthma. Sadly, 15 to 20 per cent of patients with asthma smoke and these patients are more likely to end up in hospital with acute asthma and to develop irreversible narrowing of their airways.

If you smoke, you must try to stop by whatever means you can – this requires a great deal of help from relatives and friends. 'Just the one' *will* hurt, and offering you a cigarette is a far from friendly act.

Inhaling other people's second-hand smoke (passive smoking) causes considerable suffering to children with asthma. The children of parents who smoke are more likely to have wheezy episodes and time off school than are children with non-smoking parents. This is most marked when both parents smoke, but maternal smoking seems to be more of a problem than father's smoke, primarily because most children usually spend more time with their mums.

Smoking during pregnancy increases the risk of the child being born with asthma, even allowing for all other risk factors (e.g., family history).

BREAKING THE HABIT
Any smoker who suffers from asthma should give up smoking immediately. Asthmatics should also avoid smoky atmospheres.

GAMES AND SCHOOL

Exercise-induced asthma is common in children and can cause problems, with teachers accusing kids of 'not trying' or attempting to avoid games lessons, and their own school mates teasing them for 'being useless' and other such colourful taunts. Sensible preparation can help. It is always a good idea for an asthmatic child to take a relief inhaler about 15 minutes before going out to play games. If it is used just as he runs on to the pitch, symptoms will develop before the inhaler has a chance to work.

In some children, after the first episode of wheezing with exercise, there often follows a period when they can run long and hard without problems, which may last for the rest of the session. This so-called 'refractory period' sometimes, unfortunately, has the effect of reinforcing to a sceptical teacher or schoolmate that the child was always trying to 'skive'!

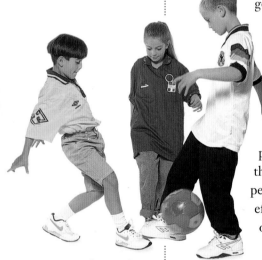

SCHOOL GAMES
A relief inhaler taken 15 minutes before any sporting activity can help prevent wheeziness.

This brings up the whole subject of asthma in the school. Many teachers are somewhat uninformed about asthma, although it must be said that they are very keen to know more if offered the chance. If you have an asthmatic child, you should take the opportunity to tell your child's teachers about the need for your son or daughter to have ready access to a relief inhaler. All too often we hear of inhalers being locked away in the school secretary's office, which may be some distance from the school playing field. By explaining to the teachers how to allow the use of a relief inhaler without permitting its abuse, the teacher's worries about the perceived dangers of inhalers will be dispelled.

SPORTS AND ATHLETICS

Many top sportsmen and sportswomen have asthma and are able to compete at the highest level. Some of the self-help advice given above for children is applicable to adults, particularly as far as use of inhalers before exertion is concerned. A warm-up period may help to some extent with the problem of exercise-induced symptoms when doing the first exercise of the day.

KEY POINTS

- Controlling house dust mites is important for some patients.
- Severe asthma may necessitate parting with a pet.
- Patients with food allergy can rarely completely control their asthma symptoms by dietary means only.
- Asthmatic patients who smoke must stop.
- Smoking during pregnancy increases the risk of the child being born with asthma.
- Parents of an asthmatic child may need to explain to teachers the need for their child to have ready access to his or her relief inhaler.

Drugs used in the treatment of asthma

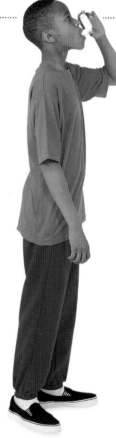

The drugs used for the treatment of asthma can be divided into three main groups: these are known as relievers, preventers and emergency (or reserve) drugs.

RELIEVERS

These drugs act by relaxing the muscle in the walls of the airways, allowing the airways to open up and air to get in and out more easily. The result is that breathing is eased. These are called bronchodilator drugs and are given in inhaled form, the inhaler usually being blue or sometimes green or grey in colour. Inhalers come in a range of different types. In most cases, inhalers should be used when symptoms occur rather than on a regular basis, although if you have more severe asthma, regular use may be needed on the advice of your doctor.

PREVENTERS

These drugs act by reducing the inflammation in the airways, thus calming their irritability. In contrast to reliever inhalers, they must be taken on a regular basis, usually twice a day. In a way, they are like a toothbrush – regular use will keep you out of trouble! Many patients keep their preventer inhaler next to their toothbrush as a

ASTHMA DRUGS
Inhalers are a convenient way of getting drugs deep into the lungs.

Inhalation of Asthma Drugs

Inhaling an asthma drug is the most effective treatment for the prevention and relief of asthma. The inhaler distributes the drug rapidly through the airways for instant relief of symptoms.

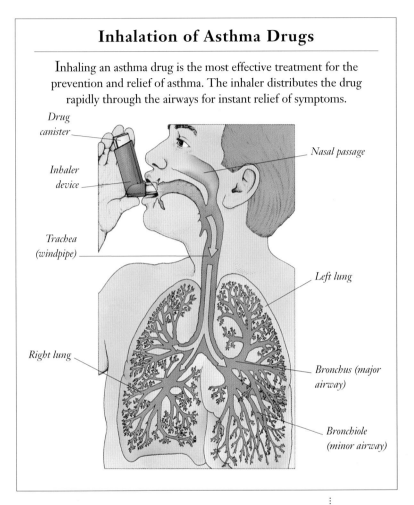

Drug canister

Inhaler device

Nasal passage

Trachea (windpipe)

Left lung

Right lung

Bronchus (major airway)

Bronchiole (minor airway)

reminder, as it can be easy to forget to take the preventer inhaler when asthma is well controlled and symptoms few and far between. Preventer inhalers are mostly brown or orange, with some red or yellow. There are three main types of preventer drug: inhaled steroids, cromoglycate (Intal) and nedocromil (Tilade). Again, these come in a variety of different inhaler devices (see pp.82–91).

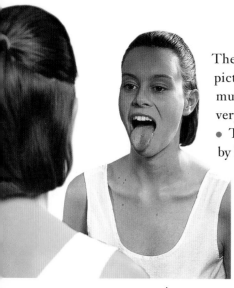

INHALED STEROIDS

The word 'steroid' conjures up disturbing pictures in many people's minds, and there is much misinformation circulating about these very effective drugs.

- These steroids are not the anabolic steroids used by bodybuilders and illegally by some athletes.

  - The inhaled version used as preventive treatment is the same sort of drug as tablet steroids used for acute attacks of asthma and, for example, in some patients with arthritis.

  - The dose of the inhaled drug is extremely small compared with that contained in steroid tablets. For instance, two puffs twice a day from a Becotide 100 inhaler delivers 400 micrograms of drug. In acute asthma, six 5 milligram tablets of steroid will be given per day – 30,000 micrograms of drug, 75 times the dose.

  - The side-effects of inhaled steroids are few compared with those of oral steroids but, most importantly, are very much less than the dangers of undertreated asthma.

  - Five per cent of patients on inhaled steroids will complain of a sore or dry mouth (sometimes this is due to thrush) while a further 5 per cent may complain of some huskiness of voice; this is more important for some patients who use their voice a lot (such as teachers or telephone operators) than for others.

  - At higher doses (1,500 micrograms per day or more), particularly in older patients, side-effects, such as easy bruising, may become apparent along with an increase in the

SIDE-EFFECTS

A few patients will experience a sore or dry mouth when taking inhaled steroids. This may be due to thrush. If you experience this, check your throat in the mirror, and see your doctor if you think there is any cause for concern.

The Main Types of Asthma Drug

- Relievers
- Preventers
- Emergency/reserve drugs

frequency of oral thrush and hoarseness. Cataracts may occur in some patients, but the suggestion that inhaled steroids cause osteoporosis (thinning of the bones) is debatable. Any such effects have to be balanced against the risks of undertreated asthma. The local effects of these inhalers can be minimised by mouth-washing after each dose and by use of large volume spacer devices (see p.46) which act as 'reservoirs' and markedly reduce the amount of drug deposited in the mouth.

The Main Types of Preventer Drug

Preventer drugs are used on a regular basis to control and minimise symptoms of asthma. This chart shows a few examples with their methods of delivery.

TYPE OF DRUG	DELIVERY METHOD
Inhaled steroids	Inhaled
Cromoglycate (Intal)	Inhaled
Nedocromil (Tilade)	Inhaled

● There is some evidence that in high doses a small proportion of children may show slight growth suppression with inhaled steroids but, interestingly, once the asthmatic child reaches adult height, growth catch-up has virtually always occurred.

Chronic, undertreated asthma of childhood is more likely to cause growth suppression than are inhaled steroids.

Inhaled steroids are very effective preventive drugs across the full spectrum of patients with asthma and are regarded as the preventive treatment of choice in most patients with asthma.

CROMOGLYCATE (INTAL)

Sodium cromoglycate has been available for as long as inhaled steroids. It is a very good form of prevention in the milder forms of childhood asthma, particularly in controlling exercise-induced symptoms. It needs to be used three or four times a day, a disadvantage when compared with inhaled steroids, but it can be used simply before exercise to prevent exercise-induced symptoms and has virtually no side-effects.

NEDOCROMIL (TILADE)

Nedocromil sodium has a preventive strength similar to that of low-dose inhaled steroids and comes as a mint-flavoured dry powder aerosol.

OTHER PREPARATIONS

There are two other groups of drugs used in the treatment of asthma, the theophyllines and the new leukotriene blockers.

- The group of tablets known collectively as the theophyllines (for example, Uniphyllin, Phyllocontin, Nuelin, Theodur) were originally used as bronchodilators but tend to be used more in a preventive way now. They are probably used less than in the past because of the effectiveness and safety of inhaled steroids. They tend to cause nausea and headache in some patients but have the advantage of being something you just swallow – some people have difficulty mastering the use of an inhaler.

- The leukotriene blockers (Singulair, Accolate) are a completely new form of asthma treatment. They are essentially preventive drugs but do have slight bronchodilator effects. Having only just arrived on the market, we are still finding our way in determining which patients may be best treated with these drugs. However, they are "tailor made" for patients with aspirin-sensitive asthma, and may prove to be the

The Main Types of Inhaled Asthma Drug

The majority of asthma drugs are inhaled. They may be relievers, which ease the symptoms once an attack has started, or preventers, which are used regularly to keep asthma under control.

RELIEVERS		PREVENTERS	
DRUG NAME	**INHALER NAME**	**DRUG NAME**	**INHALER NAME**
Salbutamol	Ventolin Salbulin Salamol Aerolin Airomir	Beclomethasone (50, 100, 200, 250, 400 micrograms)	Becotide series including Becloforte Beclazone series AeroBec series Filair series Qvar series
Terbutaline	Bricanyl		
Fenoterol	Berotec	Budesonide	Pulmicort 100, 200,
Salmeterol	Serevent		400 micrograms (inc. Turbohaler)
Eformoterol	Foradil Oxis	Fluticasone	Flixotide 25, 50, 125, 250 micrograms
Ipratropium	Atrovent Atrovent forte	Cromoglycate	Intal (puffer 5 micrograms)
Oxitropium	Oxivent		(spincaps 20 micrograms)
Fenoterol & ipratropium	Duovent		Cromogen
Salbutamol & ipratropium	Combivent	Nedocromil	Tilade

43

treatment of choice. So far, these drugs seem to have relatively few side-effects, reassuring for a tablet medication.

EMERGENCY TREATMENT

When an acute attack of asthma occurs there are two mainstays of emergency treatment available: big doses of reliever drug (often via a nebuliser) and big doses of an anti-inflammatory drug (injected or oral steroids).

Some patients will be able to self-start emergency treatment with a nebuliser and/or a course of tablet steroids, but for most patients who have not had a severe attack before, they should contact their GP as quickly as possible or attend the local casualty department. Delay can be very dangerous and it is better to be safe than sorry.

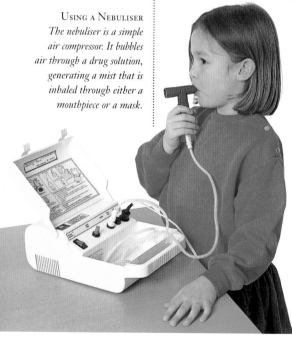

USING A NEBULISER
The nebuliser is a simple air compressor. It bubbles air through a drug solution, generating a mist that is inhaled through either a mouthpiece or a mask.

Nebulised drugs used in acute episodes are salbutamol (Ventolin), terbutaline (Bricanyl) or ipratropium (Atrovent). Nebulisers should only be obtained after assessment by your doctor. The machine itself is a simple air compressor, which bubbles air through a solution of the drug generating a mist which is inhaled through either a mask or a mouthpiece. The compressors themselves are not always available through the NHS in every health

How Drugs Act on Blocked Airways

Preventer drugs and reliever drugs act in different ways. Preventers reduce the inflammation in the airways, thus calming their irritability. Relievers act by relaxing the muscles in the walls of the airways, allowing the airways to open up.

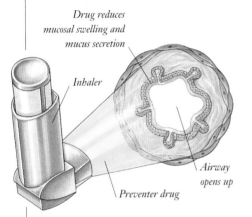

Drug reduces mucosal swelling and mucus secretion

Inhaler

Airway opens up

Preventer drug

PREVENTERS ACTING ON INFLAMED LINING

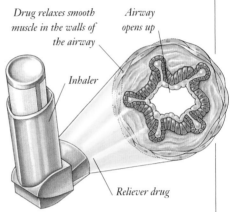

Drug relaxes smooth muscle in the walls of the airway

Airway opens up

Inhaler

Reliever drug

RELIEVERS ACTING ON CONTRACTED MUSCLE

district. You may have to buy your own or obtain one, often on a loan basis, through a charity such as the National Asthma Campaign (See p.94), whose local branches often run a nebuliser loan service.

Sometimes, nebulised drugs are prescribed to be used regularly in the more severe patient but only when high doses of other treatments have proved inadequate.

Nebulisers should not be used as an alternative to inhaled preventive treatment.

DELIVERY DEVICES

In many patients the simple metered dose inhalers (puffers) just cannot be used effectively. Poor inhaler

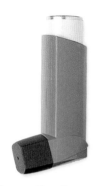

THE METERED DOSE INHALER
This device, commonly known as a 'puffer', is used to deliver fast-acting reliever drugs. Some people, particularly children, find it difficult to use.

technique can result in all the drug escaping into the air through the top of the inhaler.

The patient then believes that the inhaler is 'no good' whereas it is not being given half a chance to work. If you are one of these patients, you can use another type of inhaler device that relies on your breath in sucking the drug into the lung, as opposed to the puffer, where breathing in has to coincide with the squirt of the puffer.

The most frequently used type of 'breath-activated' device is the spacer, a large plastic balloon which acts as a reservoir of drug from the puffer for the patient then to breathe in at the right moment. Spacers are made of brittle plastic and there is some evidence that they acquire quite a lot of static electrical charge, which makes the drug stick to the inside of the spacer, thus reducing the amount of drug getting into the lungs. The best plan is to wash the spacer once a week and allow it to drip dry. Rubbing with an anti-static cloth, such as can be found in Hi-Fi shops, can also help reduce this problem.

Other types of breath-activated devices are Rotahalers, Turbohalers, Diskhalers, Accuhalers, Clickhalers and Autohalers, all of which have their benefits and

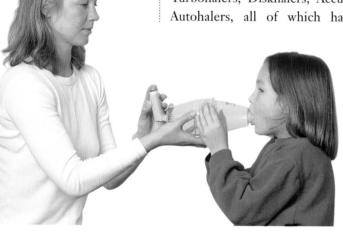

USING A SPACER
Children often find such a reservoir device easier to use than the 'puffer', as it does not require them to press and inhale at the same time. Because of its size, however, it is often a good idea for an adult to assist.

shortcomings (see pp.82–90). In many cases it is clear that an individual patient is very much at home with a particular device.

Matching the patient with the right device is vital, as an acceptable device is more likely to be used at the right time and effectively. With the exception of the spacer devices, 'breath-activated devices' are more expensive, although a correctly used 'expensive' device may, in the long term, be cheaper in terms of patient suffering than a poorly used 'cheap' device.

PHASING OUT CFC INHALERS

Metered dose inhalers (puffers) contain CFCs as a propellant. Because of the effect of CFCs on the ozone layer, puffers which contain CFCs have to be phased out. Some puffers which contain an alternative propellant have already been released and others will be on the market in 1999 and 2000. They look similar to existing puffers but tend to have a more noticeable taste. However, the drug in each inhaler is the same and they are just as effective.

KEY POINTS

- Drugs used in asthma treatment are either relievers, preventers or emergency reserve drugs.
- Inhaled steroids are the preventive treatment of choice in most patients with asthma.
- The right combination of drug and inhaler device needs to be chosen for each patient.

The management of asthma

The whole aim of managing asthma is to put you, the patient, in control of your asthma rather than have the asthma being in control of you.

In patients who require only the occasional puff of their relief inhaler, this is straightforward, but for patients with more significant asthma, guidelines – or battle plans – need to be developed and agreed by doctor and patient. Although we have already said that asthma is a very personal condition and that what is right for one may not be right for another, there are, nevertheless, guidelines that have recently been developed to help nurses and doctors in the management of all their asthmatic patients. These were developed by a panel of experts representing the different groups involved in the management of asthma.

The guidelines are simple to use but have not yet been taken up by as many doctors as we would like. They are based on a series of upward steps in treatment to control

JOINT MANAGEMENT
Doctor and patient should formulate a management plan together in order to establish good control of asthma.

48

asthma and a series of downward steps when asthma appears to be in good control and when lower doses of treatment may be possible.

Before I describe the steps, just let me remind you about the importance of preventive measures, similar to those discussed in Prevention and Self-Help (see pp.30–37), which include control of allergens. It is very important to avoid certain drugs that cause asthma or make it worse (for example, aspirin, beta-blockers). Even if you have been taking these medications for some time without problems, if you begin to develop wheezy breathlessness, stop taking these tablets. You should also stop drugs similar to aspirin, and seek alternatives (see Special Forms of Asthma, pp.61–67).

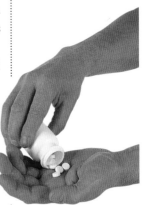

FINDING ALTERNATIVES
Some medications such as aspirin can cause or exacerbate asthma. Stop taking medications that precipitate wheezing, and consult your doctor about alternatives.

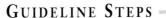

GUIDELINE STEPS

The following guidelines are the British Guidelines, recently updated, which employ a graded method of controlling asthma symptoms using the minimum amount of medication.

Step 1: Most patients fit into this level. Patients are advised to use their relief inhalers as required. If your use of the relief inhaler stays at less than one puff a day on average, no further drug treatment need be considered, although if your relief inhaler use increases you must see your doctor. If you are using one regularly more than once a day, move to Step 2.

Step 2: If you are using more than one puff a day of relief inhaler on average, you need a preventive inhaler, the choice of which is made by the doctor as a general rule (see Drugs Used in the Treatment of Asthma, pp.38–47). This should result in you reducing the use of an inhaled reliever to less than one puff a day and improvement in your symptoms.

Step 3: If your symptoms persist, your doctor will start you on higher doses of inhaled preventive treatment or consider adding another drug. Again, these decisions need to be made by the doctor but in discussion with you, the patient, and after assessment of your particular needs.

Subsequent steps: If you are still having problems the use of even higher doses of inhaled preventive treatment, oral steroid use and nebulisers, among other treatment options, will be considered. At this stage it is likely that you will be referred to a chest consultant for assessment, but we like to think that up to this step you will be managed by your general practitioner.

Step down: In medicine it is sometimes perhaps too easy to start a new treatment when symptoms do not come under control. It is not so easy to stop a treatment either because symptoms are well controlled or because the new drug had no extra benefit.

MANAGEMENT PLANS

One way of giving you particularly good control over your asthma and its treatment is to provide you with a management plan. This is a series of instructions on what to do when your asthma starts to slip or in situations in which your asthma may be thought likely to worsen. There are two types of management plan.

Steps to Asthma Control

These simple guidelines, developed by doctors and nurses involved in the treatment of asthma, allow for the minimum dose of the appropriate drug to be given so that the symptoms are adequately controlled.

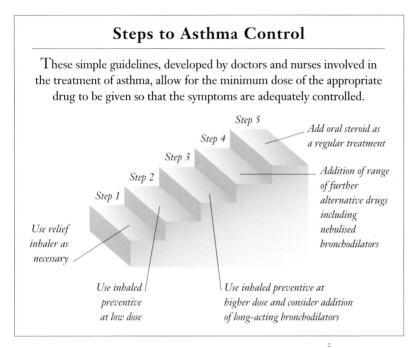

Step 5

Step 4

Step 3

Step 2

Step 1

Add oral steroid as a regular treatment

Addition of range of further alternative drugs including nebulised bronchodilators

Use relief inhaler as necessary

Use inhaled preventive at low dose

Use inhaled preventive at higher dose and consider addition of long-acting bronchodilators

PEAK FLOW-BASED MANAGEMENT PLANS

The peak-flow meter is simple to use and to read. A short sharp blow will record the maximum rate at which air can be blown out of your lungs. Usually, three attempts are made, and you record the highest. Recording a value twice a day (on waking and on going to bed) is usually sufficient, although sometimes your doctor will ask for more frequent recordings.

With a peak flow-based management plan you will be provided with a peak-flow meter, a chart on which to record the peak-flow readings, along with target values.

The first value is the target peak flow, which is usually 70–80 per cent of best. If your peak flow is above this value, you need not adjust your treatment, but if your peak flow falls below this over a 24-hour period, you should double your inhaled preventive treatment until your peak flows have climbed above the target peak flow and remained there for two or three days.

The second value is usually about 50–60 per cent of best. At this level you should use a course of oral steroids.

You may be allowed to take this course of action yourself, although some doctors prefer to see the patient if oral steroids are needed. A final threshold is that at which you should seek medical assistance as soon as possible, from either your GP or the local casualty department. This level of peak flow will be set by the doctor.

The chart for recording peak flows may either be a series of columns on which the recordings are written, usually twice a day, or a graph-like chart to plot the values. Some patients prefer this second form of chart because the variation in levels of peak flow can be more easily appreciated.

Case History 1: **PEAK FLOW-BASED PLAN**

William had always been a difficult little lad, and not just as far as his asthma was concerned. He tended to take his inhalers only when he felt the need and consequently was constantly missing school. By the time he had reached secondary school, with no sign of his asthma abating, his GP decided to try and establish a management plan.

For the first time William started to record his peak-flow readings at home on waking and on going to bed. The peak-flow meter stayed by his bed and his parents were able to check that he was recording the values on his chart. Somewhat to his surprise, William found that his peak flow readings varied considerably, dropping as low as 150 on waking but reaching 270 by evening time.

The penny having dropped, he began to take his inhaled preventive more regularly and the peak flow variation became less marked, the readings also increasing somewhat to settle between 300 and 350. By that stage he was taking two puffs night and morning of inhaled steroid and had begun to use the relief inhaler much less frequently.

The GP then gave him a target of 275, advising him to double his preventer if the values dropped below this over a 24-hour period and keeping at the higher dose until he was above target for at least three days.

A second threshold was given of 175, below which William knew to contact his GP for a course of oral steroids. In the event, oral steroids did not become necessary. William began to notice the benefits of his regular preventive therapy and over the subsequent year had to increase his inhaled steroids (when peak flows fell below 275) on only three occasions.

SYMPTOM-BASED MANAGEMENT PLANS

The same concept as that of a peak flow-based plan operates here except that certain levels of symptoms are used as prompts for changes in treatment as opposed to changes in peak flow.

Case History 2: SYMPTOM-BASED PLAN

Jacky had not got on well with peak-flow measurements. They did not seem to tell her much more about her asthma than did her symptoms and they began to be a pain to do, being 'just for the sake of the doctor', as she saw it. Luckily, the GP became aware of this and suggested a switch to a symptom-based plan. By doubling her inhaled preventive if she used more than three puffs of relief inhaler a day over two successive days, or when she started a cold, or if she started to wake at night with symptoms, her asthma was more effectively controlled. If doubling the inhaled preventive didn't stop her symptoms Jacky knew she had to go to her GP for reassessment, although if she had to do that she did measure her peak flow a few times before the consultation 'just to see'. This helped the GP believe that she was managing her asthma sensibly.

SPECIALISED HELP
Many doctors' practices now have a fully trained asthma nurse to advise asthma patients and manage the treatment of their condition.

CHOOSING A PLAN

Some patients seem better suited to peak flow-based plans, others to symptom-based plans, and the decision which to use is often based on a number of factors. Sometimes a combination of symptoms and peak flow can be used for certain individuals. Both plans will include advice to anticipate problems such as colds or exposure to known allergens. If you develop the early symptoms of a cold you should double your inhaled preventive treatment for at least a week until the symptoms pass, when you can resume the original dose. Some patients only need inhaled steroids for colds, and they should start at the slightest beginnings of a cold and continue for two weeks unless their asthma still continues to cause problems, in which case they should stay on their preventive treatment and contact their GP.

CLINIC NURSES

Asthma clinics have been set up in many GP surgeries, run either by the general practitioner or by the practice nurse. Many are run by nurses who have been specifically trained in the management of asthma at recognised training centres. Their role in the management of asthma is very important and they have helped provide a much better service for the asthmatic patient in general practice, with fewer referrals to hospital from practices where such a system operates and more appropriate referrals when there are problems.

Often, the asthma nurse will see patients with asthma more than the doctor will, releasing the doctor for other patients, but the nurse knows very well when the doctor needs to see the patient if things are not going well. It ought to be the aim of all general practices to set up an asthma clinic run by a fully trained asthma nurse.

KEY POINTS

- Guidelines have been developed to help nurses and doctors provide optimal management of all asthmatic patients using a series of treatment steps.
- One way of giving patients good control over their asthma is to provide them with management plans.
- Management plans may either be peak flow based or symptom based.
- Many GP surgeries have set up asthma clinics, often run by specially trained asthma nurses.

Asthma in elderly people

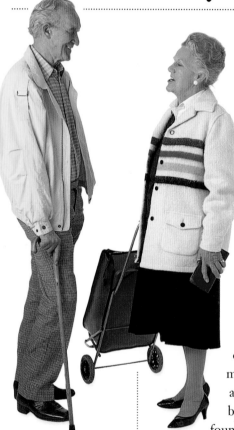

Asthma tends to be regarded as a condition of the young, particularly children, and indeed it is very much more common in children, as we have seen. As these patients become older, some have persistent symptoms, some have only minor symptoms and some have shed their symptoms to all intents and purposes.

There are some patients who develop asthma for the first time in their later years, often to their great irritation. It is often believed that these patients are more likely to have more severe asthma and to have to take oral steroids. It is also believed that allergies are less likely to be found. While these beliefs are true up to a point, it is important to realise that there is always a great overlap in patterns of asthma throughout the ages. Yet again, it bears repeating that each patient needs to be assessed as an individual.

LATE DEVELOPMENT
Although asthma is much more common in children and the young, it can persist, or even begin, in later life.

56

SYMPTOMS

The symptoms in the older patient are identical to those found in the younger patient with asthma except that breathlessness, especially on exertion, is quite common. This is often due to the fact that many folk over the age of 60 have, at some stage, smoked cigarettes and are left with a bit of irreversible bronchial tube narrowing. This means that exertion will cause breathlessness more quickly in some individuals.

Problems can occur when an older patient complains of chest tightness on exertion. As heart disease is common in this age group and angina can cause this very same symptom, delay in diagnosis – both of angina and asthma – can occur.

Case History: LATE-ONSET ASTHMA

Tom, an 82-year-old man, went to his GP with a six-month history of episodes of breathlessness. Sometimes these came on out of the blue and sometimes when he exerted himself. He did not feel that he was wheezy but did admit that he got a tight feeling in his chest, particularly when he got breathless on exertion.

Quite rightly, the GP's first impression in a gentleman of this age was that this was likely to be due to heart disease, but treatment for angina had no effect. He was sent to a consultant at hospital who felt that late-onset asthma needed to be ruled out, although he was fairly certain that this was an unlikely diagnosis. To the consultant's surprise and delight, the peak flow readings recorded assiduously by the patient showed the typical variation seen in asthma, and prescription of anti-asthma medication resulted in great improvements in his symptoms.

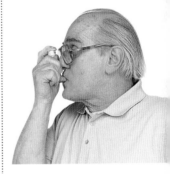

INVESTIGATING SYMPTOMS
Breathlessness in the elderly is often caused by heart disease, so the symptoms should be investigated. In Tom's case, measurements of peak flow showed that he was in fact suffering from late-onset asthma. Inhaled anti-asthma medication relieved his symptoms.

The patient's reaction on realising he had asthma was interesting in that his major reaction was one of anger.

'Why me? I've never smoked and always looked after myself. There's no one in the family who has suffered from asthma. Why me?'

Explanation and reassurance and the fact that on two puffs twice a day of inhaled steroid he improved greatly did relieve his anger. He is now able to garden as he did before with only occasional need to use his relief inhaler.

WHAT IS THE TREATMENT?

Again, treatment of asthma in the older patient with asthma is the same, and follows the same steps, as in the younger patient. Where problems can occur is in the manageability of the inhaler devices. The Rotacap dry powder system can be very fiddly for an arthritic hand and even the metered dose inhaler (puffer) can be impossible to use by patients with stiff or painful hands.

Attachments are available to make the puffer usable by these patients (e.g., Haleraid, made by Allen & Hanburys and available on request from chemists), but often a large volume spacer will ease the problem. It is really a matter of tailoring the inhaler device to the patient.

As age creeps up, patients often find themselves on a variety of different pills, potions and other medications for a range of conditions. This can often be very confusing and it is incumbent on the doctor to keep the 'regimen' of treatment as simple as possible. It may even be necessary to sacrifice the ideal treatment just to ensure that the most important treatments are taken.

Side-effects of any form of treatment are more common in the older patient. In the more severe asthmatic the side-effects of oral steroids can be severe, particularly osteoporosis and the skin changes, with easy bruising, skin thinning and poor wound healing. Patients taking high-dose inhaled steroids (more than 1,500 micrograms per day) can also develop these skin changes, although to a less dramatic degree.

WHAT IS THE OUTLOOK?

Asthma starting in later years is unlikely to leave the patient, who usually has found an unwanted companion for life. The severity does not necessarily get worse, however, and good treatment properly applied will be very effective in controlling symptoms.

Each individual will have his or her own targets or needs. For some it will simply be the ability to potter in the garden, which their untreated asthma may have stopped them doing. Others may wish to be able to go rambling again, or to be able to do their own shopping or go to the pub for a drink with their friends. Success is achieving their own target, not necessarily increasing the dose of inhaler up and up to try and achieve an improvement that the patient may not want or be realistically able to achieve.

As I mentioned earlier, deaths from asthma have increased in elderly people over the past five to ten years, but the reasons for this are not clear. I suspect that many would have been regarded as having died of bronchitis in days gone by (and, indeed, some of these deaths from asthma may be more due to chronic bronchitis today), so we must not be complacent in our attempts to prevent death from asthma at whatever age it may be causing problems.

The outlook for the older patient with asthma should be regarded positively. The treatment is safe and effective, although the more severe patient may need to find a balance between the symptoms of their asthma and the side-effects of drugs.

KEY POINTS

- Asthma can develop later in life, and these sufferers are more prone to breathlessness, especially on exertion.
- Angina and asthma in elderly people can be difficult to differentiate.
- Side-effects of asthma treatment are more common in older patients.
- Although the asthma is unlikely to go away, elderly sufferers can enjoy effective control of their symptoms with proper treatment targeted to their individual needs.

Special forms of asthma

In many cases, the cause of asthma is unknown. In others, however, an allergen will commonly trigger an attack. Other special forms of asthma include brittle asthma, aspirin-sensitive asthma and nocturnal asthma.

ALLERGIC ASTHMA

If an allergy, or more than one allergy, has been identified as being potentially important on the basis of your history, it is sometimes necessary to do further tests to confirm this and to identify the allergen. The test is simple and takes about half an hour to complete.

A series of drops of various solutions of substances, which are known to cause allergic reactions (for example, house dust mite, grass pollen, tree pollen, cat dander, etc.), are placed on the forearm. Using small needle points, the skin surface is then gently pierced through each droplet to allow the substance to get under the skin. After 15 minutes or so, local reactions can occur, which look like small areas of nettle rash and usually itch. The needle pricks themselves are not painful – just a tiny

IDENTIFYING ALLERGENS
If you suspect your asthma is caused by a particular allergen, for example cats or dogs, this can be confirmed by a special allergy test.

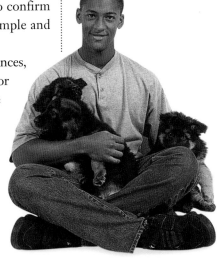

Some Potential Allergic Triggers

Asthma allergens enter the body through a range of routes – they can be inhaled, eaten or absorbed through the skin. Some of the most common allergens are shown here.

FOOD PRODUCTS

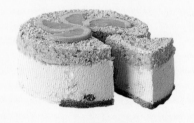

PET DANDER

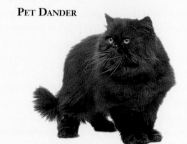

HOUSE DUST MITE

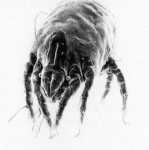

SPORE

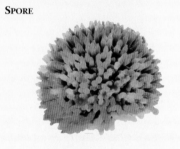

POLLEN

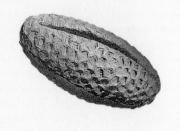

HORSE

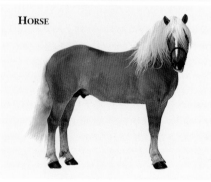

scratch – but the itching can be maddening and lasts half an hour or so.

The size of the reaction (or weal) can be measured for each allergen, which gives an idea, not only of what you are allergic to, but also how allergic you may be to each allergen. Sometimes this is helpful in management because it could tell you which triggers to avoid and could identify things which may turn out to be not so important.

The danger is that small reactions may not be very important and that patients take unnecessary actions. I have seen the occasional patient follow extraordinary and unnecessary diets, based on weakly positive skin tests, which have not helped their asthma. This is not always the case: everyone is an individual and his or her needs must be individually addressed.

DESENSITISATION

If you are shown to be allergic to a particular allergen (for example, cat or rabbit dander), if you can't avoid contact with these animals, and your asthma continues to be poorly controlled by the usual treatment regimens, then desensitisation may be considered. This should only be done at specialist centres and should only be undertaken for one allergen at a time. Certainly for patients with asthma they should be conducted only at a hospital because there have been many examples of severe reactions to desensitisation, with attacks of asthma needing hospital admission and even deaths. For hay fever alone the dangers are less, but for asthma great care needs to be taken.

DESENSITISING SUFFERERS
If you are unable to avoid contact with a particular allergen (e.g., a family pet) desensitisation is a possible option in rare cases.

The process involves a series of injections of small amounts of the substance to which you are allergic, usually under the skin of the upper arm. Very, very small quantities are used to start with, the concentrations increasing week by week to avoid severe allergic reactions. There are different time-scales over which the courses of injections are undertaken before a course is considered complete, and this will be up to the centre involved and your needs. Small local reactions (a reddening of the skin at the injection site) are not infrequent but these settle quickly on the day of the injection. Once the course is complete, boosters can be given at varying intervals if the desensitisation course has been thought successful.

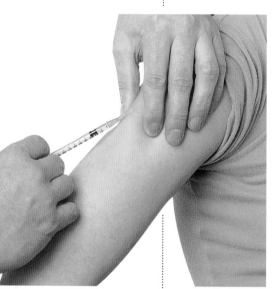

DESENSITISATION

Although rarely carried out, desensitisation involves a course of injections. Minute quantities of allergen are injected into the skin. The amount injected is gradually increased over a number of weeks until you are able to tolerate the allergen.

In the UK, desensitisation for asthma is only rarely undertaken, largely because of the fear of bad reactions, but also because many doctors do not believe that this treatment works. If you wish to talk further about whether this might be of use (and it is likely to be useful in only a minority of patients with asthma), then ask your GP for a referral to a centre with experience in this area. A list of specialist centres can be obtained from the British Allergy Foundation (see Useful Addresses, p.94).

BRITTLE ASTHMA

Brittle asthma is a rare form of asthma. The patient suffers from sudden severe attacks, sometimes in spite of apparently being very well controlled. Others develop attacks on a background of asthma, which doctor and patient have great difficulty in controlling on a day-to-day basis. These patients keep being admitted to hospital and are at increased risk of dying from their asthma.

Allergy seems to be more common in these patients and sometimes their acute attacks follow inhaling or eating something to which they are allergic. Their asthma often puts a huge strain on both the patient and family, and psychological factors seem to be very important – but whether the asthma causes the psychological disturbance or the other way around is a moot point.

Treatment is extremely difficult and patients should be managed by chest specialists with an interest in the severer forms of asthma.

CHECK THE INGREDIENTS
If you are sensitive to aspirin, be sure to check with your doctor or pharmacist before taking any medication.

ASPIRIN-SENSITIVE ASTHMA

Aspirin sensitivity occurs in around 5 per cent of adult patients with asthma, but is very rare in children. Very often these patients are negative on skin testing for allergens and may suffer from nasal polyps on a recurring basis. If you are such a patient you must avoid all aspirin-containing drugs, including a wide range of arthritis drugs such as ibuprofen, diclofenac and indomethacin. If you are unsure whether a particular drug might interfere with your asthma, ask your GP or your pharmacist. Aspirin-sensitive asthmatic patients can die from unwittingly swallowing a preparation containing aspirin.

Although the treatment usually simply involves avoidance, desensitisation can be done with success but this is only available in specialist centres.

Desensitisation for this form of asthma is done using small doses of aspirin given orally, the patient being closely monitored at hospital with repeated breathing tests for some hours after each dose. It is time consuming in the first instance but is worthwhile for some.

NOCTURNAL ASTHMA

Night-time asthma is often regarded as a particular type of asthma. In fact, waking at night with asthma is an indication of asthma that is poorly controlled overall and applies to any patient with any type of asthma. In most cases appropriate treatment will overcome the problem but some patients are more difficult to control.

In these patients, factors such as acid reflux (stomach acid coming back into the chest at night and causing irritation) may be a cause and need treatment. Some drugs, such as theophyllines and the long-acting inhaled bronchodilators, are often helpful in controlling the symptoms of nocturnal asthma.

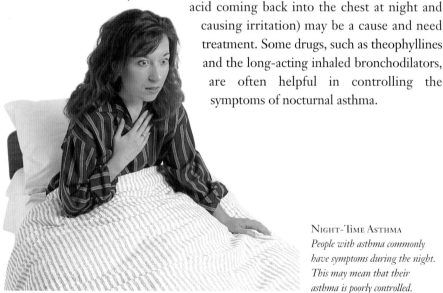

NIGHT-TIME ASTHMA
People with asthma commonly have symptoms during the night. This may mean that their asthma is poorly controlled.

KEY POINTS

- A history of allergy may lead to the need for confirmatory tests to identify the allergen.
- Desensitisation in asthma patients can be dangerous and should only be done in hospital.
- Patients with brittle asthma should be managed by chest specialists with an interest in the severer forms of asthma.
- Asthmatic individuals who are sensitive to aspirin should avoid all aspirin-containing drugs. Ask your GP or pharmacist if you are in doubt.
- Night-time asthma suggests that asthma is poorly controlled.

Occupational asthma

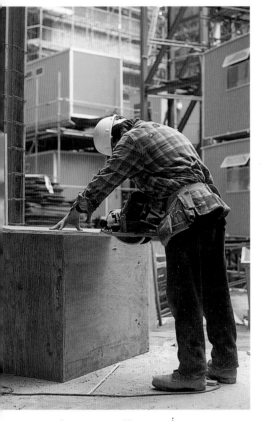

OCCUPATIONAL HAZARDS
Work that involves constant exposure to dust or another allergen can cause asthma in susceptible people. Protection may be possible, or it may mean a change of job.

Asthma that develops as a result of exposure to a substance or substances at work is regarded as occupational asthma. The exposure may act as an inducer of asthma, where the substance sensitises the patient to such an extent that further reactions are caused at every subsequent exposure.

Alternatively, the substance may act as a trigger, inducing attacks in patients who already have asthma, which did not necessarily arise originally as a result of the exposure.

CAUSES

There are over 200 known causes of occupational asthma, many of them obscure, but some of them occurring in very familiar types of work. They include isocyanates (the hardener in paints used by car body paint sprayers), epoxy resins and flour (baker's asthma).

A list of the more common causes of occupational asthma is shown opposite, along with the jobs with which these substances are usually associated.

Common Causes of Occupational Asthma

Some of the most common causes of occupational asthma are shown in this chart together with the jobs in which you are most likely to encounter each substance.

CAUSES/SUBSTANCES	OCCUPATIONS
Isocyanates	Paint, varnish and some plastic workers
Colophony	Solderers
Animal urine	Laboratory workers, animal breeders
Epoxy resins	Occupations involved with adhesives/varnishes
Flour	Bakery/catering trades
Chromium	Tanning, electroplating
Enzymes	Detergent production, drug/food technology
Hardwood dusts	Millers, joiners, carpenters
Nickel	Electroplating
Dyes	Dye manufacture
Antibiotics	Drug manufacture
Grain mites	Farmers

ABSENCE FROM WORK
Symptoms that improve during breaks from work, such as holidays, only to begin again on returning, suggest that the workplace may be the cause of a person's asthma.

COMMON OCCURRENCE

Occupational asthma may affect around five per cent of asthmatics at work. This figure is approximate and is undoubtedly an underestimate of the true amount. Because patients, employers and doctors are often unaware of the possibility that occupational factors could be important, many cases go undiagnosed, which, in some individuals, may be a problem as continued exposure to certain substances can lead to irreversible changes in the airways.

DIAGNOSIS

The first clue comes from the patient's history. If your symptoms get better at the weekend or when you are away from work for longer periods, such as holidays, this suggests that something at work may be affecting your asthma. Not all who give such a history do have occupational asthma and, equally, some who don't give such a history do end up with a diagnosis of occupational asthma. However, such a history should result in referral to a chest specialist for further investigations.

After you have been referred to the hospital or chest clinic, the specialist will ask you to record your peak flows regularly, maybe as frequently as every two hours, both when at work and away from work to look for recognisable patterns of change in the peak flow readings that would support the diagnosis.

Case History: SPRAY-PAINT ALLERGY

Brian is 32 years old and has worked in the car industry for 10 years since he had a spell in the Army, where he had begun to learn his trade. For the first four years he had done various jobs around the factory, but he was switched to the paint shop at the age of 26. Although he used to smoke 10 to 15 cigarettes a day, his only problem up to that time had been the occasional bout of winter bronchitis. During the winter of 1990, he had what he thought to be another attack of bronchitis with cough and wheeze, but on this occasion the symptoms persisted and began to wake him at night. He went to his GP who prescribed Brian another course of antibiotics and told him he really must stop smoking. This had no effect and Brian's wheezing now began to be obvious on even modest exertion. The GP felt he might have asthma and treated him to some effect shortly before Brian went off on holiday at Easter 1991.

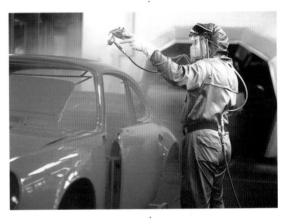

SPRAYING SAFELY
In Brian's case, a ventilated hood offered enough protection from the offending allergen – paint – to prevent his symptoms recurring.

While away, Brian began to feel very much better and even stopped using his inhalers, but as soon as he went back to work his asthma returned with a vengeance. Suspecting that Brian's improvement away from work might imply an occupational aspect to his asthma, his GP referred him to the local chest clinic where serial peak flow readings showed the typical pattern of work-related asthma. Luckily, the firm for which Brian worked was a large concern and they provided him with a very effective protective hood. Since then his asthma has been much easier to control and he has been able to continue work in a job in which he has become skilled and well paid.

CONFIRMING THE DIAGNOSIS

Occasionally, where there still may be doubt about an occupational origin for your asthma, you may be 'challenged' in the laboratory to the suspected substance under carefully supervised conditions. If you worsen when exposed to the suspect agent but not when exposed – on another day – to another substance not thought to be involved, this will usually clinch the diagnosis. This is a time-consuming process, as you may have to have a week off work, with repeated series of breathing tests being performed after differing exposures in a specially constructed laboratory. There are relatively few of these centres in the UK.

THE PATIENT'S FUTURE

Some are forced to leave their job, often because their asthma is too difficult to control while they continue to be exposed. In many cases the factory management is either unable or unwilling to improve workplace conditions. Some patients are repositioned within the company in a different job where exposure to the offending substance does not occur. Many, however, continue to work and to be exposed, which may be acceptable in some cases if their asthma can be controlled by medication. For those who are forced to leave their employment or are sacked because of poor work attendance, compensation is available for most people through the Industrial Injuries Disablement system. Ask at your Social Security Office for form B1 100 (OA) and a reply envelope, and fill in the form. More information can be found in leaflet NI 237, which can be obtained from the same place. If you have any further queries, the staff at the Benefits Agency will be able to help you.

Sometimes, claims for compensation have to go through the courts, which invariably takes time, but may be the only way a skilled worker who has lost a well-paid job can be adequately compensated.

KEY POINTS

- Asthma symptoms that improve at the weekend or during holidays suggest an occupational cause.
- The clue usually comes from the history, but the diagnosis may need to be confirmed in the laboratory.
- Compensation for those who have to leave their employment is available for most people through the Industrial Injuries Disablement system.

Complementary treatments

There is considerable interest in the role of alternative or complementary therapies for the treatment of asthma. This is due to worries about the side-effects of conventional medical treatment and a belief that 'natural substances' are better for asthma than drugs.

HEALING HERBS
The eucalyptus plant is used in herbal medicine to treat asthma.

Although virtually all of the available standard asthma treatments have been proven in properly controlled trials of efficacy, only rarely have complementary approaches been so assessed. This is why many doctors pour scorn on such forms of treatment. Yet complementary practitioners often quote anecdotal stories of benefit and maintain that consistent successes over many years show that their treatment works. This has resulted in a polarisation of belief between those who feel that conventional medicine is the only suitable treatment and those who regard conventional treatment as verging on the poisonous!

I believe that the truth lies between these two extremes although, predictably, I place more belief in standard medical treatment for asthma.

Complementary Therapies

Claims of benefit from the treatment of asthma by complementary therapies have rarely been assessed by clinical trials.

ACUPUNCTURE

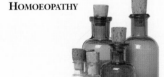

There is no doubt that acupuncture has found more acceptance in medical circles than have other forms of complementary therapy, particularly with regard to pain relief. It is also one of the few alternative approaches that has been properly tested in clinical tests in asthma. Minor benefits have been shown in mild asthma, but acupuncture has not been shown to be of help in patients with more severe asthma.

HOMOEOPATHY

There are homoeopathic remedies for chronic asthma which are claimed to work. However, the more strict homoeopaths tell me that their treatment will only be effective if the patient stops taking his or her conventional medication – something I could never condone.

HYPNOSIS

Some patients claim great benefits from hypnosis, particularly in the way they are able to cope with acute attacks or worsening asthma. For those who believe in this approach, it may be of help, but as with homoeopathy, it would be very helpful to see properly conducted trials of its effect, which, to date, are lacking.

Complementary Therapies (cont'd)

HERBALISM

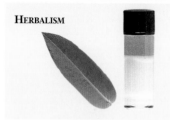

Herbalists often target their therapy on symptoms rather than the condition itself. So if cough is a predominant symptom of asthma, specific attempts to reduce sputum production will be made, often with suggestions for dietary control.

SPELEOTHERAPY

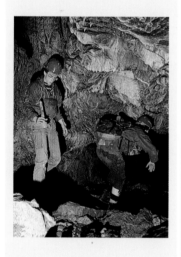

I have put this in more to make a point than to recommend it as a possible approach for the British asthmatic patient.

Speleotherapy involves patients spending time, often quite long periods, underground in caves! It appears to work, almost certainly because the patient has been removed from exposure to the house dust mite and other allergens. It is similar to the finding that spending time at altitude helps the bad asthmatic – again due to reduced exposure to the house dust mite.

So environmental control, when it involves removing the patient from exposure to allergens, can help. The problem is finding such an environment to live in!

Nevertheless, the patient needs to be regarded as a whole and not just as 'a case of asthma': his or her beliefs need to be considered and discussed and, very often, where beliefs are strongly held on both sides, compromises can be made, deals can be struck. It must always be remembered that the aim is to control asthma or at least reduce it to an acceptable level in the patient's eyes.

Conventional therapy must remain the mainstay for the treatment of asthma in the long term but in some patients who wish to explore complementary therapies, the benefits may be significant.

One important point that must be made is that patients should not simply stop their conventional treatment and switch to an alternative therapy. This has resulted in marked deterioration in some patients who have tried such a wholesale change.

Whether any benefit from complementary measures is due to an effect of belief on such a suggestible condition as asthma or to a direct effect on asthmatic airways is open to debate; perhaps that debate should be encouraged at a more scientific level than it has been in the past.

KEY POINTS

- Complementary therapies do appear to help some patients. Whether this is due to their belief in the effectiveness of the alternative approach or to a direct effect on asthmatic airways has not been established.
- With the exception of acupuncture, the benefits of complementary approaches have rarely been tested in properly controlled trials.

The future

So what does the future hold for the patient with asthma? First, there is no doubt that asthma is not going to disappear. It is very common and is likely to remain at current levels for the foreseeable future. Deaths from asthma will still occur. This all sounds very pessimistic, but there are a number of lights in the darkness which potentially hold out hope for patients with asthma.

PREVENTION

It is likely that we will become better at controlling exposure to allergens, and this will be especially important in the first five years of life, when sensitisation to the house dust mite in particular occurs. Such control will require considerable effort on the part of the individual patient or parent!

What we, as doctors, have to do is come up with a package of control measures that are practical and not cripplingly expensive. So far, we have fallen short of this ideal.

Other environmental control measures are needed, notably a reduction in parental smoking, which is so important in the development of asthma in children. There is no easy way to achieve this.

A FULL LIFE
With the new drugs and treatments available, asthma sufferers can expect to lead a fairly normal, active life.

However, there are distinct signs that pollution control measures for towns are being considered which, in time, will improve air quality and could lead to a reduction in the number of asthma attacks.

TREATMENT

Producing a drug for any new condition is a long and costly business, requiring stringent animal and human studies that have to satisfy the Committee on Safety of Medicines that the drug is both useful and safe. Only then will they provide a product licence for the drug. So what new drugs are getting through this series of hoops that might be of help to asthmatic patients in the near future?

NEW TABLETS

Interestingly, some of the new drugs on the horizon are in tablet form, as is the case with the leukotriene blockers (see p.42). After all, inhalers can be a nuisance – they are often tricky to use well and only rarely get used as regularly as doctors would like to believe.

The new drugs, whether inhaled or oral, are being studied at present and we have yet to determine whether they will benefit all asthmatics or only certain groups. Certainly, they have the potential to make asthma control easier, more acceptable and with few side-effects.

It is likely that, in the longer term, very specific treatments, perhaps aimed at particular groups of asthmatic patients, will become available.

Whether these will be in inhaled or tablet form will depend on many things, not the least of which will be what patients prefer!

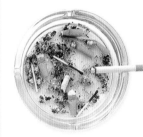

PARENTAL RESPONSIBILITY
Parents who smoke should give up the habit, as smoking has been proven to be instrumental in the development of childhood asthma.

VACCINES

The possibility of being immunised against the allergy antibody as opposed to being desensitised against specific allergens is being investigated. This sounds attractive but trials are awaited to see if this therapy is safe, practical and effective.

Immunisation against those viruses that most frequently cause asthma attacks – largely the common cold viruses (rhinoviruses) – may become a distinct possibility in the future once an appropriate vaccine, or vaccines, become available.

Again, trials will be necessary to prove that they can reduce attacks and do so safely.

GENE THERAPY

Although great strides are being made in unravelling the genetics of asthma, particularly with respect to allergy, the possibility of gene therapy is a long way off.

Potentially, this could have almost the greatest effect on asthma but there are many hurdles, both ethical and scientific, to be overcome before that time.

CONCLUSION

I am optimistic about the future for the asthmatic patient. The development of drugs with fewer side-effects or, better still, improved ways of preventing asthma or asthma attacks will come and will reduce the discomfort you and other asthma sufferers endure today.

KEY POINTS

- New drugs are being tested that have the potential to make asthma control easier, more acceptable and with fewer side-effects.
- Asthma will not be 'eradicated'; however, attempts to prevent rather than treat asthma should be effective in asthma control in the UK.

How to use your inhaler

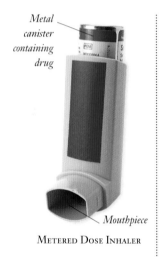

Metal canister containing drug

Mouthpiece

METERED DOSE INHALER

How to Use the Metered Dose Inhaler

1 Remove the cap and shake the inhaler.
2 Breathe out gently.
3 Put the mouthpiece in the mouth, and at the start of inspiration, which should be slow and deep, press the canister down and continue to inhale deeply.
4 Hold the breath for 10 seconds or as long as possible.
5 Wait for 30 seconds before taking another inhalation.

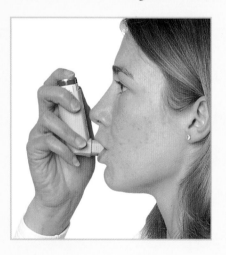

Warning

If in doubt always seek professional advice.

How to Use the Autohaler Device

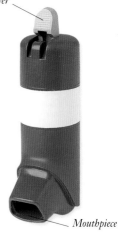

Lever

Mouthpiece

AUTOHALER DEVICE

1 Remove the protective mouthpiece cover and shake the inhaler.

2 Hold the inhaler upright and push the lever right up.

3 Breathe out gently. Keep the inhaler upright, put the mouthpiece in the mouth and close the lips around it (the air holes must not be blocked by the hand).

4 Breath in steadily through the mouth. DON'T stop breathing when the inhaler 'clicks' and continue taking a really deep breath.

5 Hold the breath for about 10 seconds.

Note: the lever must be pushed up (on) before each dose, and pushed down again (off) afterwards otherwise it will not operate.

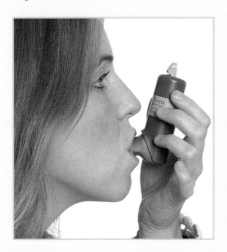

Warning

If in doubt always seek professional advice.

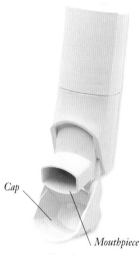

Cap

Mouthpiece

EASI-BREATHE

How to Use the Easi-Breathe

1 Shake the inhaler.
2 Hold the inhaler upright. Open the cap.
3 Breathe out gently. Keep the inhaler upright, put the mouthpiece in the mouth and close the lips and teeth around it (the air holes must not be blocked by the hand).
4 Breathe in steadily through the mouthpiece. DON'T stop breathing when the inhaler 'puffs', and continue taking a really deep breath.
5 Hold the breath for about 10 seconds.
6 Hold the inhaler upright and immediately close the cap.
7 For a second dose: wait a few seconds, repeat steps 1–6.

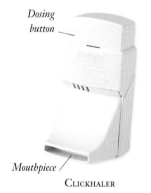

Dosing button

Mouthpiece

CLICKHALER

How to Use the Clickhaler

1 Shake the inhaler.
2 Hold the inhaler upright. Press the dosing button once.
3 Breathe out as far as is comfortable.
4 Place the mouthpiece in your mouth and close your lips around it, but do not bite it.
5 Breathe in through your mouth steadily and deeply to draw the medicine into your lungs
6 Hold your breath, take the inhaler from your mouth and continue to hold your breath for about 5 seconds (or as long as is comfortable).
7 For a second puff, keep the inhaler upright and repeat steps 1–6.

Warning

If in doubt always seek professional advice.

How to Use the Accuhaler

1 Hold the outer casing of the Accuhaler in one hand while pushing the thumb grip away until a click is heard.

2 Hold the Accuhaler with mouthpiece towards you; slide lever away until it clicks. This makes the dose available for inhalation and moves the dose counter on.

3 Holding the Accuhaler level, breathe out gently away from the device, put the mouthpiece in the mouth and suck in steadily and deeply.

4 Remove the Accuhaler from the mouth and hold the breath for about 10 seconds.

5 To close, slide thumb grip back towards you as far as it will go until it clicks.

6 For a second dose, repeat steps 1–5.

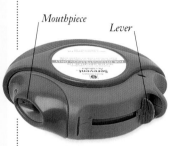

Mouthpiece

Lever

ACCUHALER

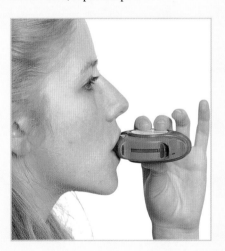

Warning

If in doubt always seek professional advice.

Grip

Mouthpiece

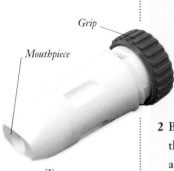

TURBOHALER

How to Use the Turbohaler

1 Unscrew and lift off the white cover. Hold the
Turbohaler upright, and twist the grip forwards
and backwards as far as it will go. You should
hear a click.

2 Breathe out gently, put the mouthpiece between
the lips and breathe in as deeply as possible. Even when
a full dose is taken there may be no taste.

3 Remove the Turbohaler from the mouth and hold the
breath for about 10 seconds. Replace the white cover.

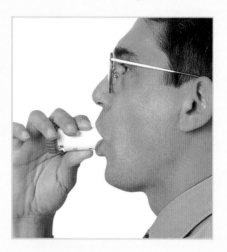

Warning

If in doubt always seek
professional advice.

How to Use the Diskhaler
To Load

1 Remove the mouthpiece cover. Remove the white tray by pulling it out gently and then squeezing the white ridges either side until it slides out.
2 Put the foil disc – numbers uppermost – on the wheel and slide the tray back.
3 Holding the corners of the tray, slide the tray in and out to rotate the disc until an '8' shows in the window.

To Use

1 Keep the Diskhaler level and lift the rear of the lid as far up as it will go to pierce top and bottom of the foil disc. Close the lid.
2 Holding the Diskhaler level, breathe out gently, put the mouthpiece (taking care not to cover the air holes each side of it) in the mouth and breathe in deeply.
3 Remove the Diskhaler from the mouth and hold the breath for about 10 seconds. Slide the tray in and out ready for the next dose.

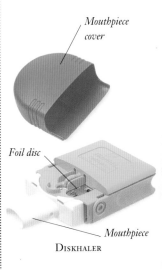

Mouthpiece cover

Foil disc

Mouthpiece

DISKHALER

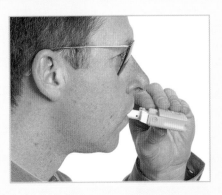

Warning

If in doubt always seek professional advice.

87

How to Use the Rotahaler

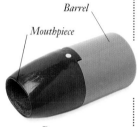

Barrel

Mouthpiece

ROTAHALER

1 Hold the Rotahaler vertically, and put the capsule into the 'square' hole, coloured end uppermost. Make sure the top of the Rotacap is level with the top of the hole (if there is already a Rotacap in the device this will be pushed into the shell).

2 Hold the Rotahaler horizontally; twist the barrel sharply forwards and backwards. This splits the capsule into two.

3 Breathe out gently. Keep the Rotahaler level, put the mouthpiece between the lips and teeth and breathe in the powder quickly and deeply.

4 Remove the Rotahaler from the mouth and hold the breath for about 10 seconds.

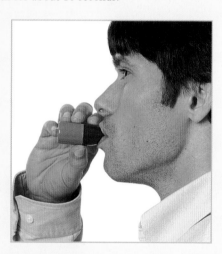

Warning

If in doubt always seek professional advice.

How to Use the Spinhaler

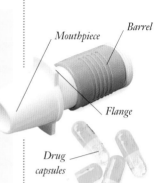

Mouthpiece · *Barrel* · *Flange* · *Drug capsules*

SPINHALER

1 Hold the Spinhaler upright with the mouthpiece downwards, and unscrew the body.
2 Put the coloured end of a Spincap into the cup of the propeller, making sure it spins freely.
3 Screw the two parts together, and move the grey sleeve up and down twice; this will pierce the Spincap.
4 Breathe out gently, tilt the head back, put the Spinhaler into the mouth so the lips touch the flange. Breathe in quickly and deeply.
5 Remove the Spinhaler from the mouth. Hold the breath for about 10 seconds, then breathe out slowly.
6 If any powder is left in the Spincap, repeat steps 4 and 5 until it is empty.

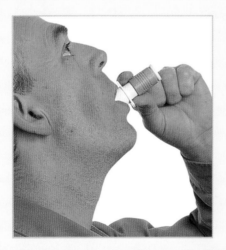

Warning

If in doubt always seek professional advice.

Inhaler slot

VOLUME SPACER DEVICE

Mouthpiece

How to Use a Volume Spacer Device

Method for patients who can use the device without help:

1 Remove the cap, shake the inhaler and insert it into the device.
2 Place the mouthpiece in the mouth.
3 Press the canister once to release a dose of the drug.
4 Take a deep slow breath in.
5 Hold the breath for about 10 seconds, then breathe out through the mouthpiece.
6 Breathe in again, but do not press the canister.
7 Remove the device from the mouth.
8 Wait about 30 seconds before a second dose is taken.

The 'Multibreath' Method

1 Follow steps 1–3 as detailed above.
2 Breathe in and out ten times using normal-sized breaths.
3 Remove the device from the mouth.
4 The next dose can be puffed into the spacer straight away.

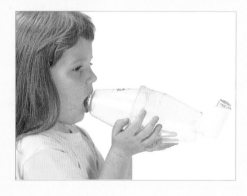

Warning

If in doubt always seek professional advice.

Questions and answers

···

Will the asthma go?

This is the question most commonly asked by parents about their child with asthma. Most children of primary school age appear to lose their asthma, often in their teens, so a condition that is more common in boys becomes slightly more common in adult women. This is not to say that the asthma has disappeared for ever, as a proportion of patients suffer a relapse in later life – in women this is often around the time of the menopause.

Sometimes, the symptoms of the newly returned asthma are different from those experienced as a child – wheezing will often be more common in childhood, and breathlessness and chest tightness more common in adulthood.

Most people who develop asthma in adult life will retain it to a greater or lesser degree for the rest of their lives. It is not clear what proportion who develop asthma in adulthood lose it, but a reasonable estimate would be around only 20 per cent.

Will the asthma or treatment damage the lungs?

Patients believe that 'the lungs' are different from 'the airways', whereas the airways are a part of the lungs.

The worry about long-term damage is, however, a real one. Undertreated, asthma can lead to irreversible narrowing of the airways because the inflammation is not being controlled. Similarly, patients who smoke and don't use their preventive inhaler regularly may develop quite severe irreversible damage to their lungs.

The treatment for asthma does not damage the lungs, although steroid tablets can cause many other side-effects, as discussed (see pp.40–42)

Taken overall, the risks of damage to the individual are greater with undertreated asthma than when the asthma is controlled.

91

Will the treatment wear off?

The drug treatment for asthma does not wear off. If you find that your relief inhaler is becoming less effective, this is far more likely to be due to worsening asthma than the drug itself having no effect. Perhaps the prescribed dose is too small or, because the airways are narrower as the asthma worsens, less will be getting to the lower airways. If you find that your treatment is becoming less effective, it is essential that you go to your doctor for reassessment. It is not true that taking a certain dose of an inhaler will lead to you needing a progressively higher dose as the years go by.

Is asthma catching?

No it is not. Asthma is not an infectious disease and cannot be caught from another person.

Are nebulisers dangerous?

A nebuliser is a powerful means of delivering drugs to the lungs and is therefore used only in the patient with more severe asthma. Nevertheless, there are some patients using nebuliser therapy for whom other forms of treatment haven't been fully explored. When used only for acute attacks,

nebulisers can save lives and admission to hospital. The danger comes when too much reliance is placed on the 'all-powerful' nebuliser and instead of seeking medical help, the patient self-administers repeated nebulised doses. This can lead to a very severe, even life-threatening, episode, which could have been avoided had the patient gone to casualty or contacted their GP.

Once a patient is established on regular nebulised therapy, clearly his or her asthma is severe. Many will never be able to stop the treatment, unless a new treatment, which may be perfect for them, comes along. Occasionally, changes in circumstances, such as a move to a different part of the country or removal from an occupational cause, can result in marked improvement in their asthma and they may then not need to use their nebuliser.

Again, as with other forms of inhaled therapy, using nebulised therapy under good supervision will not mean that you will need higher and higher doses as the years go by. If that appears to be happening it is more likely to be due to the asthma itself worsening than an effect of the nebulised drug.

Useful addresses

National Asthma Campaign (NAC)
Providence House,
Providence Place,
Islington,
London N1 0NT
Tel: (0171) 226 2260
Asthma Helpline:
(0345) 010203
This is the only charity solely dedicated to asthma. It raises funds for research and is the biggest contributor to asthma research in the UK. It has an active network of local groups run by asthmatics for asthmatics who provide a variety of services to their local population apart from raising remarkable amounts of money for research. The NAC was formed by the amalgamation of the Asthma Society and the Asthma Research Council.

The British Allergy Foundation (BAF)
30 Bellegrove Road,
Welling,
Kent DA16 3BY
Tel: (0181) 303 8525
This organisation was founded in June 1991 by a group of leading medical specialists determined to improve the awareness, prevention and treatment of allergy. The BAF encompasses all types of allergy and aims to offer information and support to sufferers, as well as raising funds for allergy-related research. Work is mainly funded by voluntary income and a small government grant towards the cost of maintaining the Allergy Helpline.

The National Asthma and Respiratory Training Centre
Atheneaum,
10 Church Street,
Warwick CV34 4AB
Tel: (01926) 493313
Fax: (01926) 493224
This centre was established as a result of the need for increasing the ability of GPs to manage asthma without referring to hospital. The centre trains nurses to manage asthma in the general practice and chest clinic setting by a combination of a distance learning package and a residential course. Their results have been phenomenal in improving the quality of asthma care delivered to patients today.

The British Lung Foundation
78 Hatton Garden,
London EC1N 8JR
Tel: (0171) 831 5831
This charity was established in 1985 to raise funds for research into all forms of lung disease. They also have a series of self-help groups around the country, 'The Breathe Easy Club', largely run by patients.

The Anaphylaxis Campaign
PO Box 149,
Fleet,
Hants GU13 9XU
Tel: (01252) 318723
For information on peanut/food anaphylaxis (that is to say, immediate allergic reaction)
(please send an s.a.e.)

Index

Acknowledgements

PUBLISHER'S ACKNOWLEDGEMENTS
Dorling Kindersley would like to thank the following for their help
and participation in this project:

Editorial: Nicola Munro; **Design:** Adam Powers; **DTP:** Rachel Symons;
Consultancy: Dr. Sue Davidson; **Indexing:** Indexing Specialists;
Administration: Christopher Gordon.

Organisations: St. John's Ambulance, St. Andrew's Ambulance
Organisation, British Red Cross.

Photography: (p.24, p.30, p.64, p.80, pp.82–91) Paul Mattock;
Illustrations: (p.8, p.17, p.45) Philip Wilson; **Picture research:** Angela Anderson;
Picture librarian: Charlotte Oster.

PICTURE CREDITS
The publisher would like to thank the following for their kind
permission to reproduce their photographs. Every effort has been made
to trace the copyright holders. Dorling Kindersley apologises for any
unintentional omissions and would be pleased, in any such cases, to
add an acknowledgement in future editions.

Richard Gardner p.55; **Pictor Uniphoto** p.71, p.76.